We would like to thank all the people who contributed their stories and reflections: service users, carers, students and qualified nurses. In particular, this book is dedicated to the memory of Janine and June. We are also grateful to all those who helped bring the updating of this book into being, including Kath McCourt, Margaret Rowe, George Philipson, Karen Heslop, Mark Cavanagh and our families and friends for their love and support. We are indebted to the team at Pearson for their constructive guidance, patience and encouragement.

We have changed the names of people in the stories to maintain confidentiality but they will recognise themselves. We would also like to thank the reviewers for their helpful and constructive comments that have helped shape the book.

Contents

Foreword

Nursing is a great profession. It is challenging, varied and interesting, offering excellent opportunities across the world and throughout a person's working life. It takes a special person to become a nurse; anyone who does not put patients first does not belong in nursing. For me, there is no other profession where you can touch human lives in such a close and intimate way. Whether you are assisting in bringing a new life into the world or alongside a family when a patient is dying, there is an aura of peace that nursing can deliver. Nurses are exposed to situations that no other job can ever offer. The significant impact on people's lives is the most rewarding experience a nurse can encounter.

Care and compassion are at the core of nursing. Jacqui Baughan and Ann Smith explore these fundamental attributes by utilising real-life examples from everyday practice settings. Students, learners, qualified nurses, carers and users of services have all contributed and shared information and reflections as a basis for exploration and analysis of nursing practice. When a person embarks on a career in nursing, they see themselves as always doing good for others. However, it is not easy. Nurses need to think on their feet, make appropriate decisions and find acceptable solutions. The sequence of chapters and true-life vignettes will take the reader on a supreme journey of highs and lows, providing knowledge, attitudes, nursing interventions and constructive reflections.

This book is a rich resource and can be revisited on numerous occasions as career challenges align with your personal and professional growth. It offers an important, creative approach to understanding more about the nature and development of compassionate nursing care, at a time of particular pressures and changes in the health-care sector. The use of real-life stories from practice is a compelling way of demonstrating that caring must be sustained at the very heart of nursing. Nursing is an art and a science born out of caring and nurtured in practice: a privileged profession.

Professor Kathleen McCourt, FRCN
MEd, BA (Hons), DipN (Lond), Cert Ed
RGN RM, RCN T, RNT

Dean
School of Health, Community & Education Studies
Northumbria University
Newcastle upon Tyne

Preface

We are very grateful to have been given the opportunity for updating this book. As the profession enters a new phase in its development as an all-graduate nurse workforce, nurses must find ways in which they can integrate increased academic knowledge and high-level skills within compassionate care delivery. The increasing scope and sophistication of modern health care are putting extra demands and strain on care and compassion in health-care systems all over the world. The effects of these are seen in persuasive stories in some of the reports and media coverage concerning shortcomings in care. We need to face issues related to the capacity for nurses to continue to care with compassion, if this is not to be lost within shifting professional boundaries, organisational change and increased public expectations.

In the pressurised and rapidly changing world of health care it is therefore important for nurses to maintain and extend their capacity to be caring through new ways of partnership working with service users and within multi-professional and multi-agency teams. The notion of compassionate caring is still seen to be at the very heart of nursing, but attempts at defining this by using rhetoric that is either too simplistic or very difficult and abstract may confuse rather than enlighten. We have therefore drawn on our long experience in practice and nurse education to write a book which is grounded in the reality of everyday practice. We did not expect to arrive at an all-embracing definition but would like readers to see the book as a means for embarking on a journey of exploration to uncover indicators of some of the many dimensions of caring. We believe that an effective way to do so is to use stories from practice as a focus for reflection. We were very fortunate and privileged that student nurses, qualified staff, service users and carers gave us their rich and engaging stories as a basis for our exploration. Without these, the book could not have been written and we owe the contributors our deep appreciation and gratitude. We have changed the names of people in the stories to ensure confidentiality but they will recognise themselves.

The stories from students and qualified nurses helped us to identify significant caring moments in practice that occurred not only in busy traumatic periods but also in everyday situations. Other stories from people about their lived experiences of illness or disability, in being cared for or providing care, helped us to identify important indicators of caring partnerships. They helped us to recognise the significance of nurses and other professionals being only one small part of a continuum of care.

The first five chapters of the book are concerned with the nature of caring relationships and provide indicators of attitudes, knowledge and nursing interventions that assist or that can be detrimental to care partnerships and therefore to effective and therapeutic care provision. Throughout the book there are reflective exercises that are aimed at helping readers relate to their own experiences but also utilise important academic and practice knowledge gained from a variety of sources. The focus of the book changes slightly in Chapters 6 and 7, where there is more emphasis on what nurses might do to recognise and increase their capacity for caring and build and maintain caring communities. In the final part of the book we review what we have learned from the caring indicators. These are summarised in Chapter 8 within the BOND framework as a means of further reflection on the nature of caring with compassion.

In the final chapter the importance of continuing the journey of identifying, implementing and evaluating dimensions of compassionate caring is emphasised and also the role of organisations in nurturing and valuing the emotional and social capital nurses bring to care. We found the stories we used both awe-inspiring and humbling. We hope you will find the same and that you will continue to see your own stories and those of your colleagues and patients/clients as a rich resource for your future personal and professional development.

In summary, this book is about the art of caring with compassion in nursing practice. It will be useful for both students and qualified nurses to help them to consider their practice and for mentors, preceptors or supervisors who support students and colleagues. Those wondering whether to embark on a career in nursing, and support workers, who are such an integral part of health and social care teams, may also find it helpful.

Jacqui Baughan and Ann Smith
June 2012

Acknowledgements

We are grateful to the following for permission to reproduce copyright material:

Text

p. 11, excerpt from Eliot, T S (1963) 'Little Gidding' in *Four Quartets*, reprinted by permission of Houghton Mifflin Harcourt Publishing Company (US rights), copyright © 1942 by Eliot, T S and renewed 1970 by Esme Valerie Eliot; excerpt from 'Little Gidding' in *The Wasteland and Other Poems* by Eliot, T S, published in 2002 reprinted by permission of Faber and Faber Ltd; p. 35, from Redwood, S (2004), Case study 3: Careers in nursing research. In: Freshwater, D and Bishop V (eds), *Nursing Research in Context. Appreciation, Application and Professional Development*, p. 130–131, reproduced with permission of Palgrave Macmillan; p. 45, excerpt from Smith, S (1981) 'Not Waving But Drowning' by permission of the Estate of James MacGibbon; p. 143, adapted from McKergow, M and Clarke J (2005), *Positive Approaches to Change: Applications of Solutions Focus and Appreciative Enquiry at Work*, with permission of Solution Books.

In some instances we have been unable to trace the owners of copyright material, and we would appreciate any information that would enable us to do so.

Chapter 1
Creating a caring discourse

Introduction

In this chapter, we introduce storytelling as a means of discovering what caring is all about. We show how theories can be beneficial and exciting in helping us to shed light on our experience and that of service users and their families. Our discussions lead to new meanings and understandings – in other words, they help us to create a caring discourse and add to the evidence base for nursing practice. From those discussions we begin to identify caring indicators, which we use and extend in later chapters to uncover a framework for caring. The overall aim is to strengthen the way to care in practice.

We discuss ways in which you, as a student or registered nurse, can make a valuable contribution to the creation of a caring environment. We will look closely at the notion of compassion in caring, the complexity of caring and the potency of a nursing presence. We consider ways in which nurses are able to 'connect' with patients and the long-lasting impact of emotional feelings. We discuss how nurses and service users can use and share stories as an important basis for reflection and also as ways of identifying key indicators of caring or uncaring practice.

Is caring still at the heart of nursing?

Do you see caring as at the very heart of what you do as a student or registered nurse? It was probably the most important reason that brought you into the nursing profession in the first place. Indeed, its importance has been emphasised throughout the profession's history. One of the most influential writers on the subject has been Watson (1985, 1999, 2000, 2007), an academic who has analysed the nature of caring and the therapeutic relationship in nursing over a number of years. However, in spite of much writing on the subject and genuine concern to be caring and compassionate, you may well think that your acts of caring are under pressure in a health-care system that has made increasing demands on you. Recently there has been an increase in adverse public outcry about the quality of care provision in the UK (Francis, 2010). In 2007 the Nursing and Midwifery Council (NMC) recognised the need to respond to public and professional concerns by including care, compassion and communication amongst its Essential Skills Clusters which had to be integrated into every pre-registration nursing programme (NMC, 2007; 2010). Approaches such as this can help us to understand the expectations of our patients and clients, and to gain the skills and qualities necessary for providing quality care. We still feel, however, that a deeper understanding is needed about the nature of, and barriers to, caring at a time when compassion is perceived to be in decline. A reflective exploration of its many different aspects and presentations, including the management and monitoring of care, will assist us even further in achieving this. The purpose of this text is therefore to determine how a greater understanding can directly inform our actions.

We begin by considering the term 'patient', which we use interchangeably with 'service user' throughout this text, primarily for simplicity. However, we acknowledge the emotion a word can bring. For example, Spencer et al. (2011) highlight problems with 'patient' and its association in many people's minds with passivity, the sick role and disempowerment. They suggest that it seems at odds with rhetoric about the importance of patient empowerment, the expert patient and the activated patient and they note that other terms such as 'client', 'customer', 'consumer', 'service user' and 'expert by experience' have also been used.

> 'Though service user is currently in vogue, its shortcomings are now being articulated, especially in the fields of social work and mental health. For example, it defines a person by a single narrow aspect of their life (using a specific service), it neglects those who do not or cannot access services, and it does not devolve power or respect to the people who use services.' (Spencer et al., 2011:13)

According to these authors, language is important because it transmits values and beliefs and can influence our perceptions and also power relationships. It is therefore is an important consideration within our discourse on the nature of caring and we will come back to its importance in Chapter 6.

We have called this chapter 'Creating a caring discourse', which is our way of summarising what we see as an exploration through storytelling of what caring really means to us as nurses and to our patients and their families. We all tell each other stories about what we feel about various situations encountered at work. In these stories we express our emotions, thoughts, knowledge, judgements, ideas and values. In other words, like us, after a hard day's work, you probably have the need to go through your highs and lows and let off steam with someone you trust. It is these stories that make up a shared nursing discourse. For example, think of the ways people using social networking sites have developed their own discourse or the way adolescents talk to each other, which is obviously very different from the way they might talk to their parents! In our work, there are also patient/client discourses and medical discourses. In this text we are using stories from people who have been involved in providing or receiving care to help create a caring discourse. The stories will be used as triggers for our discussion and we will draw on academic and other literature to gain more insights and to broaden and deepen our understanding.

We are drawing on experience gained over a number of years during which we have been studying the subject of caring by collecting critical incidents (written and verbal accounts of significant events) from patients, students and registered nurses. Some of these are quite painful and reflect 'uncaring' behaviour. Recent reports such as the Mid-Staffordshire Inquiry (Francis, 2010) and that of the Health Service Commissioner for England (2011) have led to strong reaction in the media and understandably from patient support groups, with improvement in the quality of care becoming the focus of government reports advocating reform (Care Quality Commission, 2011; NHS Future Forum, 2011) Accounts of profound deficiencies in care are a cause for concern and are distressing. They point to a need to understand not only why nurses are being portrayed as uncaring and lacking in compassion but more importantly, why this kind of behaviour might occur and how it can be prevented.

A timely reminder is contained in the NHS Constitution (Department of Health, 2012:2), which sets out the key principles and values upon which the NHS is based:

*'**The NHS belongs to the people.** It is there to improve our health and well-being, supporting us to keep mentally and physically well, to get better when we are ill and, when we cannot fully recover, to stay as well as we can to the end of our lives. It works at the limits of science – bringing the highest levels of human knowledge and skill to save lives and improve health. It touches our lives at times of basic human need, when care and compassion are what matter most.'*

Dickson (2008) notes that given the size and complexity of the health service, examples of bad care are not surprising but asserts that care and compassion must still be at the heart of nursing, however busy and complex the situation. We have found indications of immense feelings of guilt and frustration expressed by nurses if they feel that opportunities to engage in meaningful relationships with patients and relatives are thwarted. As the profession enters a new phase in its development as an all-graduate workforce we must find ways in which to enable high skills and compassion to coexist both in our own care provision and in the methods we use to support, guide and monitor others who provide care.

In our rush to get through our everyday work, we may forget that it is in very simple ways that caring can be expressed. Have you thought about the contribution those with very little experience can play? Let us consider a message sent by a relative to staff about the care her grandmother had received from Jo, a student nurse in her first placement.

Case Study 1.1

'From a relative's point of view with absolutely no experience of hospitals I didn't have a clue where to go for advice, who to ask for information or what jobs each person I came into contact with did. Jo was wonderful because she was approachable. I used to visit Gran twice a day and whenever Jo was around she would have a chat with Gran. The chat might just be, "Hello Alice. How are you today?" But she never walked by without saying something, which meant that Gran and I got to know her. Although I knew that Jo was a student and as such had no authority I realised very quickly that if I asked her something she would find out the answer and let me know as soon as possible. I felt that some of the more senior members of staff were too busy to deal with what they considered to be "trivial" questions. Jo treated my gran the way she would treat her own gran and nothing was too much trouble for her.'

Whether you are a student or a qualified nurse you may remember such experiences when you have been singled out for a particular mention in a 'thank you' card or in verbal communication, but have you considered in detail why this happened? You may almost have taken this as nice to know but not particularly significant but reflecting back on it could increase your ability to pinpoint what you did that was particularly valuable (the often hidden or 'taken for granted' aspects of nursing) so that you can use opportunities to repeat these sorts of actions in the future. You can increase your caring and skills of compassion even more if you use academic knowledge in this reflection. This is what evidence-based practice is all about. Our discussion below will help us to demonstrate this by reflecting in more depth and exploring Jo's contribution to the quality of Alice's experience of care.

Using theory to understand practice

The caring behaviour of the student was recognised and appreciated by both Alice and her granddaughter. Jo, inexperienced and in her first placement, conveyed warmth and interest, ensuring that both perceived they were important to her and that what they asked was of consequence. In short, the student was sending out a powerful message – that she cared – and she did so by using her natural warm, informal communication skills, which are an important part of social exchange. The contribution student nurses make to creating a caring environment is not a new discovery but can be found in studies of nursing practice: e.g. Morrison (1994:91) noted that students were 'singled out for their attentive care and devotion' and thought their constant availability was particularly appreciated by the patients.

Student nurses have excellent opportunities in all branches of nursing to provide holistic care and make real efforts to listen to and attend to individual needs. It is sad that the more experienced and qualified health-care professionals can sometimes be so preoccupied with competing demands on their time and energy that they may not be so easily available for providing the kind of contact that service users and their carers seek. Although students are in a position where they can develop close relationships with patients and relatives, there is a difficulty in that because of their lack of nursing experience, they may not always know how to respond effectively in complex situations (Dowling, 2006). Sadly, it could be that when opportunities for assessing and attending to individual needs arise, all grades of nursing staff fail to take them. There have been charges that some highly qualified nurses (and also some students) may be missing out on opportunities to engage in caring activities that may occur whilst providing intimate or fundamental care. It has been argued that core nursing tasks have been devalued (highlighted in the 'Too posh to wash' debate (Wright, 2004) and have led to a rise in concern related to what is described as 'basic' nursing care (Francis, 2010). It is said that nurses have distanced themselves from these, focusing instead on high technological or management roles and target-driven priorities. Indeed, according to

Youngson (2008) the increasing scope and sophistication of modern health care are putting a strain on care and compassion in health-care systems all over the world.

Although organisational and economic pressures and skill-mix decisions may have resulted in fewer opportunities for 'hands-on' care, it is reassuring that some experienced nurses such as Freshwater and Biley (2005:14) have questioned the assumption that nurses think themselves too superior to undertake such tasks, saying that '. . . our own experiences as nurses on a variety of busy wards were quite the opposite. We enjoyed being able to escape to the patient; those hours spent behind the curtains managing "basic care" provided the ideal opportunity to engage in what was for us central to nursing: the therapeutic relationship.' It may be, therefore, that if compassion is to be the cornerstone of care, it is imperative that registered nurses continue to have opportunities for providing this, and of being role models for others. Sadly, although the centrality of caring to nursing has been there since the profession was established, it seems to be the one thing that might be so easily lost, diluted or undervalued as other priorities take precedence.

Time to think back

+ What do you think?
+ Do you think you make the best of the opportunities when you help patient/clients with fundamental care needs? Are they able to talk about their fears and concerns?
+ When you delegate fundamental care to others, how to you monitor the quality of that care in terms not only of the completion of the task but the ways in which it was carried out? Do you include the patient or carers in that evaluation?

Students and health-care support workers are important resources. Valuable communication exchanges between patients and relatives and qualified staff may be affected by restricted opportunities, professional status and demanding role responsibilities. As we have seen in Jo's story, patients and relatives may be anxious not to burden more senior staff with what may seem to them to be 'less important' matters so instead they may approach the student or support worker. The relationship Jo had with Alice and her granddaughter was helpful and supportive, benefiting from the opportunities they had to become familiar and comfortable with each other through the informal social exchanges that took place during their encounters. Ersser (1997) has described the value of 'natural' emotional exchanges. Students often see the worth of these forms of communication when they begin their careers and perceive these 'natural' emotional exchanges as an essential component of being able to 'care'. Being able to help people is, for most, the main reason for coming into nursing in the first place and becoming 'distant' is what many say they are most fearful of (Smith, 2003).

An added problem is that the very nature of caring in a compassionate way may not be well understood, as we shall go on to examine in the rest of this text. Caring may be taken for granted as something that comes naturally, particularly for women, but its complexity (for example, the emotional as well as the physical skills required) may be underestimated (Smith and Gray, 2001). Compassion is an integral part of this and if nurses are to give effective patient-centred care of the kind we would want the closest members of our families to receive, we need to look for ways in which this is demonstrated.

Looking more closely at compassion in caring

Consider the following story to gain insight into how a patient might experience compassion from a student nurse. Harry, a 50-year-old businessman, described his hospital experience:

Case Study 1.2

'I was in a medical ward after a heart attack. I've always felt in control of situations and hated being ill. I think I coped with this by making myself the life and soul of the ward. I'd chivvy up the other men and we'd have a laugh about what was happening to us like going to X-ray wearing backless nighties! When my family and friends came in we'd talk about football and what was going on "outside". I talked to my wife about the tests and treatment and she spoke to the doctors and nurses. When she was there I did my best to make everything seem normal. One night I woke up and couldn't get back to sleep again. Rashida, a student nurse, noticed I was awake and asked me if I wanted a cup of tea. When she brought it, she must have noticed something was wrong because she asked me how I felt and for some reason I started to cry. I couldn't stop and I felt so stupid.

I said to her, "Everyone thinks I'm coping but I'm not!" She just sat and held my hand. I told her that I didn't want my wife to know that I wasn't really a strong person. It's hard to know how long I wept but it seemed as if she sat with me for a long time and not only then but several nights after she would come and sit with me for a while when it was quiet in the ward and we'd talk about how I was overcoming some of the fears I had of dying and leaving my family. I'm very appreciative of all the care I had – you couldn't fault the medical care I was given. I had full explanations of everything but when I look back I still remember that time in the middle of night and how much that student nurse's presence meant to me.'

To think about

+ Think about what we can learn from Harry's story about the nature of presence as part of compassion.
+ Think about a situation in your practice. Reflect on how your presence has helped someone who was frightened or anxious. This might be a patient or a relative.

You might want to record this within your Ongoing Achievement Record (OAR) if you are a student or Continuous Professional development (CPD) profile if you are a registered nurse. Remember to use pseudonyms to protect patient confidentiality.

Harry's story helps us to understand the importance of holistic care and shows that the emotional features of care are as important as the rest of the knowledge and skills required to care. It illustrates how important it is to be 'available' to give supportive care (not just technical care), and to have a 'caring presence'. This is what can be described as showing compassion. It also demonstrates the opportunities for care which nurses working at night can have. Kirby and Slevin (1992:73) cite Marcel, who, writing in 1949, spoke of the nature of real presence:

> 'The person who is at my disposal is the one who is capable of being with me with the whole of himself when I am in need; while the one who is not at my disposal seeks merely to offer me a temporary loan raised on his resource. For the one, I am a presence, for the other, I am an object.'

Harry did not feel he was treated as an object. We can infer this because he was able to tell the student nurse of his fears. Perhaps this was easier for him to do than to tell his wife because he would have been less worried about upsetting her. Rashida was able to show that she cared only because she spent time with Harry, held his hand and waited for him to talk but she also followed this up by being available on subsequent occasions. These may only have been for a few minutes but would have made Harry feel that his feelings continued to be seen as significant and he would have felt more comfortable with his disclosures.

Roach (2002:28) has helped to deepen our understanding of the nature of human caring and describes caring as a natural capacity of human beings. She emphasises that it is 'not an exceptional human quality, nor the response of an exceptional few . . . It is the most common, authentic criterion of humanness.' This is perhaps why students, even with little professional experience, can be so good at it. Roach (2002:71) reaches the conclusion that people use occupational roles to express their natural, and self-fulfilling, human capacity to care. She describes this as the core value since 'it inspires, directs and sustains nursing's identity and the identity of all persons who choose professions of care'.

Rashida entered nursing with a really useful resource – the capacity to show compassion. The important issue to consider is how we use our 'natural' human capacity to care within our practice and also what may stand in the way of how we can develop and extend it. It may not be as straightforward as we may initially believe. There is some evidence that health-care students rethink their notions of caring soon after they enter the professions, and this questioning of their fundamental beliefs causes them uncertainty and doubt (Clouder, 2005). Other studies indicate that nurses feel disillusioned following qualification. Maben et al. (2007) noted the frustration and 'burn-out' newly registered nurses experienced as they found they were unable to provide what they most wanted to give: patient-centred, holistic care. The authors found that this led to 'job-hopping' and in some cases a decision to leave the profession. It would seem therefore that for the sake of the quality of service we provide and the future of our profession, more knowledge of how caring and compassionate attitudes and approaches are maintained, whilst working within complex and demanding health care systems, is imperative.

The complexity of providing care

The nature and value of nursing have been debated in all branches of the profession. It would seem surprising that there has been a long debate about the relative value of skills in technical tasks as opposed to those of being engaged in fundamental care. It is interesting that Tarlier (2004) believed that this kind of debate about the relative importance of different caring skills has stopped productive discussion and, rather than helping, has taken place at the expense of understanding the complex nature of nursing.

To think about

+ Think about your care of a particular person.
+ What caring skills were you using?
+ Do you think some were more important than others?

You will find your answer will be influenced by a variety of factors, depending on the urgency of the situation, the most pressing needs of the patient/client or their families, and so on. Reflecting back on the situation, were there any other caring skills you wish you had used?

Did you find it difficult to say that one skill was more important than another? If you had asked your patient, would you have got the same answer? It is therefore also a question of who is making a judgement about what was important about the care. Patients or relatives may have a very different perception of the situation. Youngson (2008), an experienced anaesthetist by profession, reflected on his experiences when his 18-year-old daughter was hospitalised with a life-threatening condition. He stresses that 'Few hospital patients ever remember what was said to them, or what was done, but the emotional experience is lived for a lifetime.' Therefore, the debate about the relative importance of each skill has little validity but uncovering the dimensions of compassionate caring will help us more in our understanding of what effective, holistic caring is all about. In other words, we are searching for what puts the caring into care.

As nurses, you will be aware of the high emotional feelings that caring for someone can bring and may sometimes have wondered whether you responded in the best way. Have you ever been left feeling uncomfortable, challenged and emotionally, as well as physically, drained? On the other hand, have there been times when you found your nursing experience very exciting and interesting and you have gone home feeling that you have done a good job? Perhaps these highs and even the lows contribute to make nursing one of the least boring and most rewarding jobs.

As we have discussed, to unravel the complexities of what we mean by caring practice, there is a need for a degree of reflectivity or time to mull things over. Over the past few decades much emphasis has been put on reflective practice within the context of holistic, individualised care often described as the ideology of nursing practice (ideas of what nursing is or should be). This kind of care brings with it many challenges. Each individual is unique and has distinctive physical, psychological, social and spiritual needs. For example, try to imagine a situation in which a young man called Jimmy Jones is admitted to an accident and emergency department (A+E) with a paracetamol overdose and a diagnosis of alcohol abuse. A holistic caring approach will consist not only of managing the serious life-threatening event but also of finding ways of providing ongoing help in such a manner that Jimmy feels recognised and valued as a human being in every interaction with health-care professionals. This will need the integrated, thoughtful, patient and non-judgemental approach of an interdisciplinary team.

Nurses contribute to the care within an effective team. Good nursing care calls for a complex mixture of ingredients - the combination of experience, knowledge and skilled practice - but it also depends on motivation and enthusiasm. In Jimmy's case, excellent holistic care requires the application of a range of knowledge (for example, amongst other things, the science of the human body, the psychology of dependency, legal aspects and ethical frameworks) and practice skills (assessments and interventions likely to overcome a life-threatening event, risk assessment and a range of longer-term interventions). But these alone do not make care complete. Knowledge and skills need an essence of caring applied in an artistic way such as through the use of empathy and self-awareness and perhaps creative responses to meet individual needs. We think that this sort of care is what people mean when they say that good nursing combines both art and science which creates a feeling in the recipient that someone has gone that 'extra mile for them'. It is what changes a good nurse into an exceptional nurse.

> *The authors of the NHS Constitution (2012) highlight the importance of the necessity of providing a compassionate approach to skilled care. It states: 'We respond with humanity and kindness to each person's pain, distress, anxiety or need. We search for the things we can do, however small, to give comfort and relieve suffering. We find time for those we serve and work alongside. We do not wait to be asked, because we care.'*

Dunlop (1986) describes this kind of caring as a public form of private love and it may well come close to the rewarding aspects that many nurses entering the profession say they hope to experience. It would seem, however, that special experiences of care may not be related to dramatic and unexpected events, but instead be an integral part of an everyday experience in which patients' needs are really met.

The potency of the nursing presence

We have already seen how the presence of both student nurses, Jo and Rashida, demonstrated caring communication and compassion and was a powerful or potent influence. There are times, however, which unfortunately we all come across, in the hustle and bustle of everyday practice, in which some caring aspects are missing. Consider the following story given to us by Julie, a relative, and think about why she was so upset. What did one nurse do that made all the difference?

Case Study 1.3

'My mother was seriously ill and although we felt that the nursing staff were polite, they gave us minimal attention and information and we thought that they were not really wanting to listen to us. I guess they might have believed they were giving good enough care but to be honest, it wasn't really good enough for us as they were not really available and seemed to be avoiding us. One evening when we were feeling particularly despondent, a bank nurse came into the room. She stood for a moment and then asked us how we were and how Mum was. It was the first time we felt that someone cared and really wanted to help. This gave us the opportunity to say what we were worried about – which was how Mum's pain was being managed. The outcome was that within hours a Macmillan nurse came and Mum became pain free for the first time for days. Thank God for that nurse!'

From Julie's story it seems that in general the nurses' world of care was far removed from what Julie and her mother needed. The nurses focused on what they perceived as the pressing activities and may even have thought that they were giving good care, or they were so immersed in the ward routine they weren't thinking about individual patient needs. It is interesting that in telling her story, Julie saw as particularly significant the action of the bank nurse who 'stood for a moment'. This nurse gave the impression of availability. She was summing up the situation and was in a state of readiness to listen. That simple act made all the difference in the implementation of effective care and it is this kind of action that we need to consider and extend. These examples are in line with Barker's (2003:9) suggestion that an important way of considering care is with an emphasis on 'caution, attention to detail and sensitivity that is necessary when handling something precious'. He draws parallels with the work of an archaeologist who adopts a *care-ful* strategy for unearthing and revealing a possible find, including sensitivity and attention to detail.

Actions may be unthinking if they are part of routinised procedures. The actor and playwright Alan Bennett (2005:12) wrote about the impact on him of what he describes as 'the casual cruelties that routine inflicts' when visiting his mother who had just been admitted to a psychiatric unit. 'She had on admission been bathed, her hair washed and left uncombed and uncurled, so that now it stood round her head in a mad halo, this straightaway drafting her into the realms of the demented. Yet the change was so dramatic, the obliteration of her usual self so utter and complete, that to restore her to even to an appearance of normality now seemed beyond hope. She was mad because she looked mad.'

These stories point to the problem of dehumanising routines and chaotic ruses of activity and preoccupation, both of which lead to loss of individuality and a danger that patients and their relatives or friends feel they are overlooked or ignored. A nursing presence is likely to provide a potent caring indicator in that the nurse acknowledges the intrinsic worth of each individual.

Time to think back

So far we have uncovered indicators about what Alice, Harry and Julie saw as important aspects of caring and also what they saw as unhelpful. We can use these positive indicators as pointers or signposts to guide us on our journey in creating a caring discourse. For example, we saw that just being there and being emotionally available can significantly improve patients' and relatives' experience of care. You will uncover more indicators through reflections on more stories as you progress through the text and we will use these to gain a fuller picture of the components or dimensions of caring. Since reflection is such an important part of this process, we will spend a little time looking closely at how we can use stories for this purpose.

Using stories to create a caring discourse

Stories create vivid images that remain with us and help us to learn. We know, from our own and others' experiences, that we repeatedly recall certain specific moments that have had an impact on us. You will have recounted these moments as stories, or anecdotes, to others because they are meaningful to you. In simplistic terms, we reflect back on our experiences. As Schon (1983) notes, this is 'reflection on action' and in your nursing programme you will be directed to using reflective models as a means of helping you to learn most from particular situations that have occurred in practice. Stories help us to look again at a situation and find new meanings and understandings. Our nursing students have found a quotation from a poem by T S Eliot (1963:222) very useful in summarising the impact of new discovery within a familiar situation:

> 'We shall not cease from exploration
> And the end of all our exploring
> Will be to arrive where we started
> And know the place for the first time.'

We can use stories as the means for furthering our journey of exploration into caring and because stories are an important part of everyday life – they form a vital way of communicating with and relating to each other. We hear stories every day in our workplace and they can have an important impact on our individual practice. What we learn from them may guide and influence us in our ways of working as well as our beliefs, values and expectations. However, if we use these stories without reflecting on them, we may build up nursing myths, some of which may be helpful and some less so, e.g. the myth that nurses should not become emotionally involved. By using stories as a focus for our reflection we can critically explore myths, beliefs and values and so increase our knowledge of caring by building up a caring discourse.

Stories help us to connect one with another and so it is important that we listen and reflect on stories from those being 'cared for' (e.g. Francis, 2011). This helps us to become more knowledgeable about their perceptions of the caring process and so be in a better position to learn from and transform nursing care. We have to be sure that the resulting discourse is one in which questioning occurs and assumptions are challenged and one way of achieving this is through shared, critical discussion that may need courage at times (Firth-Cozens and Cornwell, 2009).

Phillips and Benner (1994:vii) reiterate the importance of sharing caring narratives that help us understand good practice. 'We believe it is essential to recover the vision of what is possible in actual practices today.' These nursing academics think that through the knowledge gained by sharing actual experiences we will able to have a greater impact on future policies and decisions about how care is provided. This emphasises the importance of sharing and learning from experiences – so something we may undertake on a daily basis can be turned into a truly learning exercise.

Reflections can be about happy experiences and moments that have made us feel successful and competent. However, there may also be times when we are anxious, shocked, sad, angry, guilt ridden and fearful and when we are greatly puzzled by our own and others' responses, leaving us with unanswered questions. You are likely to encounter a number of these moments in nursing and you may tend to share these experiences with individuals who are important to you, perhaps colleagues who understand you and with whom you feel safe. On the other hand, there are times when you may have difficulty in discussing them for a variety of reasons. You may think that others will judge your thoughts, questions, feelings or actions since in sharing something personal we put ourselves at risk of judgement. Stories, therefore, have another important feature that needs to be taken into consideration.

The way we tell and reflect on our stories depends on who is listening to us. As Mishler (1991) says, any story is socially reconstructed and reflects the content and the expected audiences. A case in point: your reflections as part of your educational course or in clinical supervision are likely to take on a different form from 'storytelling' occurring with a colleague in an informal setting. Whatever form it takes, however, we can learn from storytelling. Stories are linked with our self-image, or ways in which we see ourselves. They help us consider the role we are 'playing' in a particular location.

Smith (2003) suggests that storytelling, as part of the reflective process, can help nurses test out possibilities for future behaviours and help refine and/or integrate ideas about various concepts. She came to this conclusion by using the research method of narrative analysis, which led her to focus on trying to discover the moral of the stories nurses told as students and as graduates: in other words, why they told particular stories in the first place. This approach helps to identify significant phrases such as the one Julie used ('she stood for a moment . . .'), which are particularly important to the individual telling the story but can easily be missed. Julie, whose mother needed pain relief, told the story because she wanted to convey the way in which the bank nurse gave time to the family and picked up their distress. The impact of changes in Alan Bennett's mother's appearance highlighted by the phrase 'She was mad because she looked mad' emphasises the impact unthinking 'routines' can make, in this case in reinforcing a stereotype. This approach points to the benefits to be gained from writing down stories and looking at them in more depth.

We have found that using written stories from students and qualified nurses has helped us over a number of years to understand practice better (Smith and Russell, 1991; 1993). We used them in workshops where participants were able to compare their hopes and fears with those of others and they also provided an opportunity for us all to gain increasing awareness of what can inform and influence future nursing practice.

The importance of using stories from service users and carers has also become increasingly recognised. The online Patient Voices Project is 'to facilitate the telling and the hearing of some of the unwritten and unspoken stories of ordinary people so that those who devise and implement strategy in health and social care, as well as the professionals and clinicians directly involved in care, may carry out their duties in a more informed and compassionate manner' (**www.patientsvoices.org.uk**). The stories provide powerful, honest and moving insights into the varied experiences of patients and carers, including descriptions of their emotional and physical challenges, fears and concerns. The presentation of these in a digital form provides a useful way of learning about and from these experiences, access to which is often missing in more formalised educational or care situations.

Stacey and Hardy (2010) utilised a method of learning gained from the Patient Voices Project by asking newly qualified nurses to tell stories about the challenges they faced in the early days of their transition from student to staff nurse and to reflect on them. The digital stories they created were then used by student nurses in their final stages of a pre-registration programme, who were able to reflect on them as a group and consider ways in which they might respond in similar situations. The authors also found that students were able to learn by observing the reflection in action undertaken by the qualified nurses. They concluded that such stories were able to provide unique insights into the reality of clinical practice and create opportunities for use with mentor and preceptor presentation programmes.

To think about

Write a brief story based on an incident from your practice which made an emotional impact on you:

+ Just write as if you were telling the story to a trusted friend.
+ Underline any phrases that you see as particularly significant.
+ Think about why the story was important to you.
+ Consider what you have learned and how this will affect your future practice.

You might like to keep this as part of your reflective learning diary and/or ongoing achievement record or CPD profile.

Sharing stories with others

We have seen that sharing stories can be very helpful and this was illustrated by Vicky, a newly qualified nurse who brought the next incident to one of our reflective workshops. She wrote about an important and frequently questioned aspect, that of 'having emotions' when caring for patients. As you will see, Vicky ended her written account by wondering whether it is acceptable for a nurse to cry. She indicated that she had asked herself this question as a student but even years after it still remained an issue for her. Sharing it helped her understand the complexity of caring and why the question had remained with her for so many years. We think it is one you too may be asking yourself!

Case Study 1.4

'I was a newly qualified nurse and the consultant, the house officer and I approached an elderly gentleman called Henry who had been frequently admitted to the ward with heart failure. Henry seemed a warm-hearted man and had made an impression on me. The consultant said, "I am sorry, we have come to the end of the line; we have talked about this before, your heart is not strong enough to recover this time." I was shocked as I had not realised his heart failure was so "end stage" and that he was so poorly. The two doctors left and I looked at Henry, who started crying. What should I do?

I sat on the bed next to him and began to sob too. Henry gave me a hug. He told me that he believed in God and that he wasn't frightened of dying. I felt he was comforting me, but surely it should be the other way around? Eventually I left him. The senior nurse took me into the day room. He said it proved that I was human and that nurses have feelings. I did feel a little better, but felt that crying may not have been the best way of handling this situation. After all a nurse can't cry; can she?'

This story illustrates the uniqueness of the encounters between patients and professionals. In this instance, nurse and patient shared an intense, close and significant moment. It seems that Vicky's main focus is on finding a correct way of responding in the situation. Nurses should not cry! Nurses can cry! We think that the story illustrates the type of questions that nurses ask themselves but one to which they often fall short of finding a simple and satisfactory answer. It is difficult to articulate what is expected of a nurse, a 'caring professional'. Could it be that there is no simplistic correct answer to this and other similar questions?

Using reflection to increase our understanding

By reflecting, or looking again at the story, we can see that this newly qualified staff nurse, in trying to make sense of the situation, is unlikely to find an 'ultimate truth'. In order words there will not be one straightforward answer. This does not mean reflection is not helpful but that it helps us to come to terms with the nature of knowledge that is often incomplete and uncertain. Work by Carl Rogers (1978) might help us understand this. He suggested that there is no such thing as a static truth, but instead truth is about a series of changing approximations - we make judgements based on our varied experiences and perhaps limited knowledge.

Different perceptions and views of the same events are illustrated by the clinical psychologist Pamela Stephenson, who is the wife of comedian Billy Connolly. Pamela writes about her husband's disturbed, abusive and dreadfully poor childhood in Glasgow and notes how he survived and triumphed over this. In the introductory remarks to her book (Stephenson, 2001:1), she recalls her emotional reaction relating to the tremendous effect these circumstances would have had on him, and notes Billy's retort to her emotional response was, 'Well, I didn't come down the Clyde on a water biscuit.' Perhaps this story demonstrates that whatever events occur, traumatic or otherwise, there are different perceptions and understandings to be made about their impact and the influence they have on us. She pointedly says, 'for every one life, there are a million observed realities, including several of the subject's', so talking this over may have made them both think again and see things in a new light.

In summary, to explore the story of Vicky's response to Henry it is helpful to reflect by using a wide variety of perspectives and, in doing so, try to gain a 'best fit' understanding of the situation at hand. 'Factual' answers (answers that can be claimed to be completely scientific, objective, accurate and applicable/transferable to all circumstances) may at times be difficult to find. Although clear evidence and rational explanations have a vital role in care situations and interventions, many aspects of practice cannot be easily explained by applying a theory that covers all aspects of unpredictable human situations. We can, therefore, as an alternative, look for literature, perspectives or theories, in order to help illuminate, or shed light on, what Schon (1987) describes as the unpredictable and 'swampy world of everyday practice'.

Nursing in the dark

An early but influential qualitative study by Melia (1987) revealed some very interesting ideas about what it is to be a nurse. Her study with student nurses concluded that they learned to 'get the work done', 'learn the rules', 'nurse in the dark' and 'be professional'. Using her work can lead us to reflect on the similarities in the situation the newly qualified staff nurse found herself in, still wondering whether or not it was really all right to cry in front of a patient and speculating about what her work really should involve, trying to learn and/or remember the rules about being a professional.

This seems to be what is happening to Vicky. Whilst the incident is occurring she begins to ask herself what she should do next when Henry starts to cry. Sharing this incident with colleagues in a reflective session helped her to see that she was almost unthinkingly using good communication skills when she sat next to Henry to try to comfort or reassure him. Someone suggested that she started to sob due to a 'heavy personal attachment' she had for Henry and another questioned whether this was a good thing to have. Others disagreed and asserted that, by crying openly in front of Henry, she showed him that she cared about him and this displayed a characteristic of a caring nurse.

Most of her colleagues at the workshop thought that showing emotions as part of a caring approach is beneficial and an aspect of a therapeutic approach to care (and in written reflections later were able to draw on references in the literature to back this up: e.g. Peplau, 1952; Leininger, 1978; Barber, 1991; Ersser, 1997; Dowling, 2006).

However, as you can see in the incident, at the time Vicky felt uneasy, as if she sensed these were not, as she saw them, the 'rules' of everyday professional practice. Despite being given a form of reassurance from a more senior nurse, she continued to feel that she might have handled her emotions in this situation in a different way. In the discussion group, her colleagues inferred from her final comment, *'After all a nurse can't cry; can she?'*, that Vicky was not clear about the 'rules' in this situation. From their discussions they concluded that showing emotion is an important aspect of care but were aware that this could be overwhelming at times. Talking over the incident with colleagues and gaining perspectives from literature helped them become more aware of how common such emotions are. Freshwater (1999:29) confirms the benefits of this approach, suggesting that reflection provides an important opportunity 'for caring individuals to explore and confront their own caring beliefs and how these beliefs are executed in practice'.

We have seen the importance of reflection in increasing our understanding, so if you look for ways in which theory can help explain and analyse practice, it will not only help to ensure you keep up to date academically, but, more importantly, it will become an integral part of your ongoing development as a nurse so that the quality of the care you provide is increased. It can also help you gain in confidence. Smith (2003) found that reflection helps students and qualified nurses to become more confident in their ability to react to changing circumstances, including the ways in which they demonstrate caring. We all have a tendency to become static and unadventurous by clinging to that which we feel safe and comfortable with and so may be reluctant to reflect. Such an approach can have dire consequences for us all since without learning from the past or the present, we cannot explain what nursing is all about and we may be prone to ritualistic and unthinking care so that good care is compromised and the 'freedom' to progress is lost. We may, for example, not be aware of the importance and impact of the way in which we 'connect' with patients.

Time to think back

+ Have you ever felt out of your depth and overwhelmed in terms of your emotional response to situations?
+ Using a reflective diary might help to look again at the situation and see things in a new light, such as understanding why you felt so upset.
+ Did you cover up your feelings or did you talk to someone else? You wouldn't be alone in feeling like this. One of the skills that you need is how to handle close relationships within professional boundaries and also to help others to do so. This may be an important topic for reflection within mentorship, clinical supervision or when you are supporting and supervising other health-care workers.

Connecting with patients using emotional labour

Just like you, many nurses have meaningful moments with their patients during which a very close connection is made that may have been quite emotional. Nursing theorists, such as Parse (1992), explain the importance of patient and nurse co-creating the unique human experience of illness within a relationship of 'connectedness'. Smith (1992) captures the essence of this when she quotes a patient who praises the nurses who held her hand 'both literally and metaphorically'. However, the closeness of some of our relationships with patients and their families can seem quite challenging.

Nurses have to learn to cope not only with the task in hand but also with the emotions that sometimes threaten to overwhelm them as practitioners. A number of authors, such as James (1989) and Smith (1992), use the phrase 'the emotional labour of nursing'. The demands of emotional work can be as hard as physical and technical labour, but not so readily recognised and valued although emotional work has a key role in the creation of a caring environment (Smith and Gray, 2001).

Smith (1992) drew on the work of the sociologist Hoschild, describing emotional labour as requiring 'surface and deep acting', which nurses learn to use when there is a gap between what they do and what they feel. You may have made a determined effort to appear calm when a patient is angry or seems hostile or you may have overcome feelings when encountering distasteful smells. What you are doing then is surface acting in which you consciously change a facial expression to show a particular emotion that you want others to perceive. In deep acting we change the feelings inside us by, for example, conjuring up images, so that we show the feelings we want the other person to see. For example, we might imagine that it was our relative or friend we were caring for so that we then display more caring attitudes. Good actors are adept at intentionally manipulating thoughts, feelings and behaviour so the purpose of emotional labour and 'acting' is to produce an outward appearance that helps in the connectedness of the relationship.

Connecting with patients and being yourself

In something of a contrast to labouring with our emotions and 'acting' in response to these, another early study by Jourard (1971) is helpful to our deliberations. He asserted that nurses need to learn to 'be themselves' with patients. He said that genuineness and congruence (what is being portrayed by our actions corresponds to that which we feel internally), warmth and positive regard are important in demonstrating that we care for others. Jourard believes that nurses should find ways of expressing themselves and their emotional concerns - rather than hiding or denying them - and sums this up in his phrase 'The Transparent Self'.

Self-awareness and the therapeutic use of self are identified as key requirements for effective interactions and connectedness. To see how this relates to practice, if you return to the incident with Henry who was given bad news, we think Vicky was showing her 'transparent self', her emotional concerns were not hidden or denied, but rather 'congruent' with her behaviour. She cared about him and she showed this, but was very concerned that this was not the right way to behave, perhaps wondering if it would have been better (that is, more therapeutic) for Henry if she had laboured emotionally and, in her terms, 'acted in a more professional' manner. Probably the best answer would have come from asking Henry what his perspective of the situation was! However, we believe that this nurse was able to give Henry something very precious by caring for him in this transparent and congruent manner. This can be particularly challenging when news has to be given of unexpected deaths.

Reid *et al.* (2011:14) quote a retrospective study by Finlay and Dallimore (1991), which showed that parents were more grateful about how the news of the death of their child was communicated to them if it was undertaken by police officers than by medical staff. 'These families felt they received a greater sense of empathy from police officers, who restrained their emotions less and appeared to be visibly upset when breaking the bad news. This gave the relatives the impression that the police officers had connected to them on a personal level' (page 14).

The nature of the close or 'connected' nursing relationship and the ways in which this is managed will be an important aspect of our discussion in the following chapters. Another aspect, which we will also return to later, concerns another interesting question that Vicky asks when she wonders if it is appropriate for Henry to offer some sort of comfort to her – the 'professional'. It seems that she is expected to be the provider rather than the receiver for this relationship to be therapeutic.

Have you experienced something like this in your practice when you have been frustrated because you wanted to be able to give a 'perfect' response in an emotional situation? What we have learned is that we will rarely be satisfied with what response we give but the emotions engendered may stay with us for a long time.

The long-lasting impact of emotional feelings

Even if you have been in nursing a relatively long time, you may have expected you can still probably remember the emotions you felt in your first days in practice. Sean, who gave us the following story, says he remembers an incident vividly, even though it occurred many years ago. He is now a university lecturer and says he relates this story to students who struggle with guilt feelings and unanswered questions when they cry in front of relatives. It helps us to explore further the impact of emotional feelings concerning patients to whom we particularly connect.

Case Study 1.5

'My first post after qualifying was on a trauma intensive care unit. I was on duty one afternoon when John was admitted with severe head injuries following a road traffic accident. It soon became apparent that the injuries John had sustained were so serious he would not survive. His parents were informed of this and were obviously very upset at the news. I was allocated to look after John and his parents; they spent a lot of time at John's bedside and we talked about his treatment. His mother also asked questions about my life and during the discussion we determined that I was only four days older than John. This somehow seemed to help his mother. The following day I was again allocated to care for John. His mother brought some photographs of him and showed them to me and talked about John – what he was like, his job and his friends. Over the next few days of caring for John I felt I got to know him very well through his mother.

A few days later I came on to the ward to discover that John had died. His parents came in and his mother put her arms around me and cried openly. The emotion was so intense that I also cried. We exchanged few words, as they weren't really necessary. That night when I got home I lay on my bed and cried. I was really upset that John had died. Even though we had never spoken, the discussions I had with his mother made me feel that we had known each other all of our lives. My mother came into my bedroom and asked what was wrong and when I told her she said she could not understand how I could be so upset over someone I had never really known. I did know him, even if he did not know me!'

Sean says that he believes the incident taught him that it is important to 'be you' and not try to hide emotions. Because he behaved in a congruent manner in that his feelings and behaviour matched and he did not try to 'act the professional part' (whatever that may actually be) he showed he cared about John and his parents. Sean thinks that this helped the parents, especially John's mother, to grieve for their son. As for himself, Sean says:

> 'I often wonder what John's voice sounded like. I really felt I knew him, although I never even heard him speak. The fact that he was so close to me in age also had something to do with why his mother got close to me and I got close to John. It was as if I did know him.'

This raises an important question. Why is it that with some patients we feel as if 'a button is pressed within us' and we feel more linked into their lives, deaths, problems and issues? Fosbinder (1994) describes this as 'clicking' – an immediate rapport between patient and nurse – that facilitates the process of 'getting to know you' but can also lead to the uncovering of some deep emotions within us. Perhaps some situations may be more significant and even problematic for us because the situations somehow remind us of someone who has died or from whom we are now parted or we worry about losing someone close to us. It may also be that we become more aware of our own mortality. Reflecting back on such situations can lead us to a deeper understanding and acceptance of ourselves and others.

Summary

All these incidents, stories and scenarios are rich, potential learning experiences; they help us to connect with others and are the beginning of our journey into the development of what we hope will be a useful caring discourse. We have also discussed the importance of stories in highlighting problems in the quality of care given and the ways in which they can influence public perceptions and government reports and policies. The discourse arising from these stories has led us to raise many questions and some of the key issues such as:

+ The importance of understanding and developing the skills of compassionate caring for nurses and the impact on service users and the profession.
+ How stories can act as a focus for understanding health-care experiences, and for linking to theoretical perspectives that can provide us with an evidence base for practice.
+ The identification of aspects that are sometimes overlooked or underestimated, for example the importance of 'being there', of a caring and compassionate presence. These indicators can point us to ways in which we can improve our nursing practice.

Looking forward

We will build up a collection of such indicators at the end of each chapter. At the end of the text all these caring indicators will be used as indicative criteria for a framework of caring. This framework will help us to know more about the dimensions of a caring approach, integrating compassion, empathy, concern and kindness within a context of skilled, informed evidence-based nursing practice. In the next chapter we will continue our journey by considering what else goes on within a caring relationship by exploring what we receive from as well as what we give to these.

Activity

Look at the caring indicators. Use them as you think will be most beneficial. For example:

+ Apply them to your practice and note when you have done this.
+ Consider how your actions and reflections can help you achieve academic and/or professional requirements.

Caring indicators

1. Providing individualised, holistic care by responding to basic care needs, remembering that 'small things matter'
2. Showing compassion in actions in response to those in pain, distress, anxiety or need
3. Being approachable and comforting and making the most of opportunities to be available for patient and family
4. Communicating compassion with warmth, transparency and kindness, labouring emotionally when required
5. Being aware of how language can transmit values and beliefs
6. Recognising emotional and behavioural responses in ourselves and others
7. Listening to and reflecting on stories from those being 'cared for' in order to become more knowledgeable about their perceptions of the caring process
8. Using professional knowledge (including theories and stories from experience) to ensure practice is informed and compassionate
9. Guiding and monitoring others to whom we delegate care, helping them to demonstrate compassion and interest
10. Being aware of public concerns and keeping up to date with government and professional reports and frameworks which promote quality care

References

Barber, P (1991) Caring: the nature of the therapeutic relationship. In Jolley, M and Perry, A (eds) *Nursing: A knowledge base for practice*. London: Edward Arnold.

Barker, P (2003) Person centered care: the need for diversity. In Barker, P (ed) *Psychiatric and Mental Health Nursing: The craft of caring*. London: Arnold.

Bennett, A (2005) *Untold Stories*. London: Faber & Faber.

Care Quality Commission (2011) *The state of health care and adult social care in England 2010-2011.* London: Stationery Office.

Clouder, L (2005) Caring as a 'threshold' concept: transforming students in Higher Education into health (care) professionals. *Teaching in Higher Education* **10**, 4,505-517.

Department of Health (2012) *The NHS constitution for England (2012 edition)* London: Department of Health. Available at: **www.dh.gov.uk/nhsconstitution** (last accessed 04/03/2112).

Dickson, N (2008) Foreword to Goodrich J and Cornwell J (2008) *Seeing the Person in the Patient; the Point of Care Review paper.* London: King's Fund.

Dowling, M (2006) The sociology of intimacy in nurse-patient relationship. *Nursing Standard* **20**, 48-54.

Dunlop, M (1986) Is a science of caring possible? *Journal of Advanced Nursing* **11**, 661-670.

Eliot, T S (1963) *Collected Poems 1909-1962.* London: Faber & Faber.

Ersser, S (1997) *Nursing as a Therapeutic Activity: An ethnography.* Aldershot: Avebury.

Firth-Cozens, J and Cornwell, J (2009) *The Point of Care; enabling compassionate care in acute hospital settings.* London: King's Fund.

Fosbinder, D (1994) Patient perceptions of nursing care: emerging theory of interpersonal competence. *Journal of Advanced Nursing* **20**, 1085-1093.

Francis, R (2010) *Independent Inquiry into care provided by Mid-Staffordshire NHS Foundation Trust January 2005-March 2009.* London: Stationery Office.

Freshwater, D (1999) Communicating with self through caring. The student nurses' experience of reflective practice. *International Journal for Human Caring* **3**, 28-33.

Freshwater, D and Biley, F (2005) Heart of the matter. *Nursing Standard* **19**, 14-15.

Health Service Commissioner for England (2011) *Report of the Health Ombudsman on 10 investigations into NHS care of older people.* London: Stationery Office.

Kirby, C and Slevin, O (1992) A new curriculum for care. In Slevin, O and Buchenham, N (eds) *Project 2000: The teachers speak.* Edinburgh: Campion Press.

James, N (1989) Emotional labour: skill and work in the social regulation of feelings. *Sociological Review* **37**, 15-42.

Jourard, S (1971) *The Transparent Self.* New York: Van Nostrand Reinhold.

Leininger, M (1978) *Transcultural Caring: Concepts, theories and practices.* New York: Wiley.

Maben, J, Latter S, Macleod Clark J (2007) The sustainability of ideals, values and the nursing mandate: evidence from a longitudinal qualitative study. *Nursing Inquiry,* 14, 2, 99-113.

Melia, K (1987) *Learning and Working: The occupational socialisation of nurses.* London: Tavistock.

Mishler, E (1991) 'Once upon a time ...' *Journal of Narrative and Life History* **2/3**, 101-108.

Morrison, P (1994) *Understanding Patients.* London: Baillière Tindall.

NHS Future Forum (2012) Available at **www.dh.gov/nhsfutureforum** (last accessed 12/01/2112).

NMC (Nursing and Midwifery Council 2007) *Essential Skills Clusters (ESCs) for Pre-registration Nursing Programmes.* Nursing and Midwifery Council Circular 07/2007.

NMC (2010) *Standards for Pre-registration Nurse Education* Nursing and Midwifery Council Circular 07/2010.

Parse, R (1992) Human becoming: Parse's theory of nursing. *Nursing Science Quarterly* **5**, 35-42.

Patient Voices Programme. Available at: **www.patientvoices.org.uk** (last accessed 15/01/ 2012).

Peplau, H E (1952) *Interpersonal Relations in Nursing.* New York: Putnam.

Phillips, S and Benner, P (1994) *Crisis of Care.* Georgetown: Georgetown University Press.

Reid, M, Dowell, J and Hoskins, R (2011) Breaking news of death to relatives. *Nursing Times* 107, 5, 12-15.

Roach, M S (2002) *Caring, the Human Mode of Being* (2nd ed). Ottawa, Ontario: CHA Press.

Rogers, C (1978) *On Becoming a Person: A therapist's view of psychotherapy.* London: Constable.

Schon, D (1983) *The Reflective Practitioner.* London: Temple Smith.

Schon, D (1987) *Educating the Reflective Practitioner.* San Francisco: Josey-Bass.

Smith, A (2003) Learning about reflection. PhD thesis, Northumbria University, Newcastle upon Tyne.

Smith, A and Russell, J (1991) Using critical learning incidents in nurse education. *Nurse Education Today* **11**, 284-291.

Smith, A and Russell, J (1993) Critical incident technique. In Reed, J and Proctor, S (eds) *Nurse Education: A reflective approach.* London: Edward Arnold.

Smith, P (1992) *The Emotional Labour of Nursing.* London: Macmillan.

Smith, P and Gray, B (2001) Reassessing the concept of emotional labour in student nurse education; the role of link lecturers and mentors in a time of change. *Nurse Education Today* **21**, 230-237.

Spencer, J, Godolphin, W, Karpenko, N, Towle, A (2011) Can *patients be teachers?*
  Involving patients and service users in healthcare professionals' education. The Health Foundation. Available at: **www.health.org.uk** (last accessed 22/01/2012).

Stacey, G and Hardy, P (2010) Challenging the shock of reality through digital storytelling. *Nurse Education in Practice*, **11, 2**, 159-164.

Stephenson, P (2001) *Billy.* London: HarperCollins.

Tarlier, D (2004) Beyond caring: the moral and ethical bases of responsive nurse-patient relationships. *Nursing Philosophy* **5**, 230-241.

Watson, J (1985) *Nursing; the philosophy and science of caring.* Boulder CO: University Press of Colorado.

Watson, J (1999) *Postmodern nursing and beyond.* Toronto: Churchill Livingstone.

Watson, J (2000) Via negative: considering caring by way of non-caring. *Australian Journal of Holistic Nursing* 7, 1, 4-8.

Watson, J (2007) *Human Science and Human Theory of Nursing Care.* London: Jones and Bartlet Publishers International.

Wright, S (2004) The value of values. *Nursing Standard* **19**, 15-16.

Youngson, R (2008) *Compassion in Health Care: The missing dimension of health care reform?* NHS Confederation Futures Debate, paper 2, London: NHS Confederation. Available at: **www.debatepapers.org.uk** (last accessed 13/01/2012).

Chapter 2

Caring as a two-way process of giving and receiving

LEARNING OBJECTIVES

By the end of this chapter you should have an understanding of:

1. The benefits of rewarding partnerships in nursing care
2. What we gain from, as well as what we give to, those relationships, particularly from 'small' often unrecognised actions
3. The benefits to be gained and openness to learn (through trust and honest exchange) from patients with experience and their carers
4. The importance of promoting satisfying relationships for informal carers
5. The importance of role modelling in demonstrating compassionate care

Introduction

In this chapter we consider the satisfaction to be gained from caring for others. Early images portrayed nurses as self-sacrificing 'angels' administering to the sick for no personal gain, but changes in nursing itself and the climate of professionalism and diverse career opportunities have done much to dispel that myth. However, understandably there is still a focus on what nurses give to service users in the kind of care they do or don't provide and, less so, on what they gain themselves from their relationships and care opportunities. The purpose of this chapter is therefore to explore the nature of mutuality (what we share) and reciprocity (what we give and receive) in our caring relationships as we work towards true partnerships with service users and their carers. It will help us to understand the care relationship better and what we achieve in rewarding or 'connected' relationships. However, as a great deal of care is undertaken by family and friends in the community, we will also consider the relevance of this for them too. In this chapter, we will also return to a consideration of how we might use theory to help us explain what is going on in our working lives.

Images of nurses

Nurses have been represented in many different ways. In the past they have been portrayed as 'ministering angels' illustrated in the image of Florence Nightingale as the 'Lady with the Lamp' providing comfort and help to wounded soldiers in the Crimea. This image was one of selflessness and uncomplaining service to patients and of subservience to the medical model of care. The angel image has brought its problems in that it fails to convey the academic knowledge, critical thinking and practical skills that nursing involves. It may also lead to unrealistic expectations. 'If nurses are angels,' suggest Summers and Summers (2010:195), somewhat scathingly, 'then perhaps they can care for an unlimited number of patients, though research shows fewer nurses means higher patient mortality.' Other media images such as the 'dragon matron' and the 'sexy female nurse' also continue to portray nursing in a particular light and are still influencing public perceptions, in spite of more recent attempts to overcome the stereotyping and portray a more skilled and professional image.

Since the 1960s there have been massive scientific and technological changes in the nature of health care and the volume of activity within hospitals and community settings in the UK. Alongside this has been the development of nursing knowledge and skills, reflected in changes in nurse education at both pre- and post-registration level. The increased requirements in clinical, academic and organisational skills have, not surprisingly, led to the implementation of an all-graduate workforce in the UK. However, some of these changes appear to have been counterproductive in terms of public trust in where nursing is heading, particularly following adverse publicity from the reports by Francis (2010) and the Health Service Commissioner (2011). There are fears that nurses are no longer at the bedside but instead there are images of nurses as 'uncaring' and 'lacking in compassion'. The growth of patient advocacy groups using the internet has added to the debate. An example of this is the 'A dignified revolution' website, which was begun in 2008 to improve the care of older people in hospital. In its discussion of the reason for setting up the group the authors assert: 'Many nurses provide outstanding care. However, the attitude and behaviour of some nurses when caring for vulnerable older people does not reflect the duty of care that they have towards their patients. The experience of many of those involved in A Dignified Revolution is that some nurses do not consider that basic nursing care is part of their role. Instead, they consider it is the role of the healthcare assistant.' (**www.dignifiedrevolution.org.uk**)

This is an important point and needs to be taken seriously since according to the Department of Health (2008) patients and relatives see nurses as the 'owners' of the caring system. However, Robertson (2010) argues that linking examples of lack of care to academic progress in the profession is unfounded.

'Critics should also remember that times have changed. As well as being compassionate, modern nurses must be able to lead teams, analyse data and manage complex care. The role has changed and so the training should too. Being able to provide patients with good quality care does not mean compassion is any less important. [. . .] Many other caring professionals, such as doctors and physiotherapists, are trained to degree level without being tarred with the same brush. Prospective nurses, like other degree-educated health-care professionals, enter the profession because they genuinely want to help and care for others. To say that because they have a degree they are unable to care is simply illogical.'

We will go on to consider the challenge of providing compassionate care and the barriers to this in Chapter 3, where we discuss the evidence and possible reasons for poor care and ways we might ensure it does not occur, but for now it is useful to remind ourselves of how much we gain from the recipients of the care we provide.

Perhaps you recognise this in your own experience in which your interactions with a patient or his or her family helped to make you feel good. For example, someone may have given you a special 'thank you' or even a word of encouragement when you were having a bad day. At a time when morale may be low, it becomes increasingly important to give and receive thanks from our colleagues. This is more likely to foster a culture in which compassion and empathy are promoted. It will be useful if you continue to think about this as we move on in our exploration of caring because we see nursing care as a series of partnerships – in which we give but also receive. When we feel we are doing a good job and others recognise it, we get a boost to our self-confidence and gain the satisfaction of knowing that we are helping others. Perhaps, though, there are days when things do not go so well. Can you think of times when you have been despondent and felt like a 'spare part'? This often happens to students when they begin their nursing programme and see everyone else looking as if they know what they are doing. However, it is a common experience and may occur throughout your professional life as you meet new challenges and develop your practice-based knowledge. It is reassuring to know that as your experience grows so too does your ability to adjust to and learn from new challenges.

Moving towards a rewarding partnership

Consider the following story told to us by Marjorie, a community nurse. Think about how she was able to turn a 'spare part' experience into a positive one, beneficial for both Sukwinder (the patient) and Marjorie herself.

Case Study 2.1

'Sukwinder had recently returned home from hospital following treatment for metastatic breast cancer. As her community nurse I visited her regularly, monitoring her symptom control, liaising with her general practitioner (GP), arranging for the installation of equipment and helping her to apply for state benefits. However, she appeared to be an organised, self-reliant individual. I began to feel that once the practical issues had been sorted out she did not really need me. I knew she had a strong informal support network as well as close links with the Macmillan nurse, the hospice and the hospital. Perhaps she considered me to be yet another cog in the wheel of the health service that she had to endure because it is the system. I felt increasingly uncertain about the value of these visits. Could it even be that my visits were detrimental to her well-being as I was a reminder of her illness and a disruption to her everyday life? Should I withdraw temporarily?

But despite my misgivings I continued to visit. One day when I arrived, she was resting on the settee and complaining that her legs were swollen and heavy. Without really thinking about what I was doing, I knelt down and put my hands on her feet. They felt so cold. I instinctively started to rub her feet gently in order to warm them a little. I asked her if she had ever had a foot massage. She said, "No, not really but I like having my feet played with!" So I just rubbed and stroked her feet. At intervals she talked a little.

After twenty minutes or so when I had finished, Sukwinder asked me if I would have time to do it the next time I came. I felt good about myself. I felt that I had eventually been able to do something to make her feel better.'

Time to think back

+ Have you ever found yourself in a similar situation or feeling irritated or frustrated because you never seem to be able to help some people enough?
+ Do you agree that Marjorie believed that it was important that whatever care she gave was seen as beneficial and valuable by Sukwinder? It was therefore a process not just of giving but also of receiving something in return, an acknowledgement that what she did was helpful and therefore provided positive feedback which made her feel good.
+ Can you apply this to the situation you thought about when you felt awkward or out of place?

You will be aware that not everyone makes us feel valued. Some people seem to make 'demands' on our time or are even hostile towards us. They may be doing so in response to their situation and we have to ensure that because we do not find it easy to care for them or they value us less, we do not ignore them, avoid them or treat them unprofessionally. We will consider these difficult kinds of situations further in Chapters 3 and 6 but for the moment we will stay with the importance of feeling valued.

Achieving a connected relationship

In the story, Marjorie, the community nurse, was almost instinctively able to use an opportunity that presented itself. If she had given up and withdrawn initially, this would not have happened. Sukwinder gave her the opportunity to care both then and in the future. According to Roach (2002:68), the connectedness of a relationship does bring with it certain responsibilities on both sides: 'Whenever we are in a relationship with another person, we establish bonds and these bonds, grounded in trust, entail duties and responsibilities – an ethic of relational responsibility.' What Roach is emphasising here is the importance of acknowledging that there are expectations on both sides of any relationship. In applying this to nursing, it is useful to consider what we expect from service users. These may be emotional gifts such as recognition of our capabilities, our skills and our qualities, or, perhaps, a positive response to our suggestions or advice – all the 'feel good' factors gained from having been a help to someone else. We may also gain other gifts such as learning opportunities and even reassurance.

Marjorie's story also demonstrates other important aspects of relationship building. It shows that if nurses concentrate only on negative features, such as the things they may feel unable to do or situations in which they perceive their ability to contribute is very limited, there is a danger that they may ignore positive aspects. It shows that by relaxing and having an open and friendly approach, nurses may find new opportunities that they might miss if they are preoccupied with only doing or saying 'the right thing'. Perhaps in our drive to be seen as highly skilled practitioners, we forget about the value that basic human warmth and presence can bring, particularly in undertaking small acts. Smith (2008) highlights the importance of the 'small things' such as ensuring that spectacles are clean, dentures are in, hearing aids are operating and hair washed. Barker and Davidson (1998:351) also stress the importance and benefits of this for mental health nursing:

'What little evidence exists suggests that when people become psychiatric patients, they would rather receive care than some sophisticated therapy; they require valida-tion of their experience rather than processing for change; they desire an encounter at a fundamentally human level, rather than a carefully negotiated . . . consumer–provider contract.'

Vivien Lindow (1996:186) (who is a service user herself) reinforces this by writing about the difficulties people with mental health problems have communicating with professionals:

'One of the most persistent complaints about service users is "They never listen." But diagnosis and the effects of psychoanalysis get in the way of listening. The medically inclined listen to the words of service users in order to diagnose: "Is she psychotic?" This robs our words of their meaning. The analytically inclined listen to demonstrate their skill in gaining insights. This again robs our words of their meaning. If we dis-agree with our clever analyst (or even therapist or counsellor) it demonstrates denial, projection, transference or one of the other 'mechanisms' that stop what we are com-municating to be heard.'

We have to be careful that we do not resort to using professional jargon as a way of explain-ing and justifying our interventions. We also need to be aware of what is called the 'impact of meta-communication', which demonstrates the complexity of communication and why it can so easily lead to problems. Using the example above we can illustrate this: Lindlow is thinking about what the professional is thinking about her thinking. She suggests that is problematic because the professionals are using their own various frameworks as explanations rather than listening enough to her. The complexity of communication is an area that causes most problems for service users in all areas of health and social care (Health Service Commissioner for England, 2011) so there is a need for ongoing professional development about this impor-tant topic area . It seems that establishing partnerships with service users that are built on trust and honest exchange can be difficult since many other aspects, such as professional knowledge, expertise and an unequal power relationship, may (although we may find them helpful) cloud perceptions and even get in the way of clear and effective communication.

To think about

Think carefully about Vivien's story and what we can learn from it for practice:

+ Think about how the way you communicate can cause problems for service users and their families.
+ Think about your own area of nursing. You may be caring for adults, children and young people, or for people with learning disabilities. How is Vivien's experience applicable to your area of work? Do we sometimes jump to the wrong conclusions?

You might like to keep this information as part of your reflective learning diary/ongo-ing achievement Record (OAR) and /or professional development portfolio.

Using theory to help us explore the nature of patient–nurse relationships

We can expand our discussion about how we might achieve and maintain effective partnerships further by considering a study that was undertaken over a decade ago but from which we can still learn a great deal. This may help us to recognise and respond to those relationships that may cause problems.

Theory helps us to think about aspects that we might not otherwise consider. Morse (1991) undertook a research study of a variety of care situations from which she was able to describe two main types of patient-nurse relationships: mutual or unilateral. The first type she called mutual relationships, which differ in terms of involvement and intensity and depend on a number of factors such as the length of time they occur, common needs and desires, and personality factors. These relationships are partnerships and mutually beneficial. There is a general agreement in terms of what is expected of each other and the kind of behaviour that may occur. However, the unilateral, or one-sided, nurse-patient relationship, is characterised by asynchrony (people are out of step with each other) and this kind of relationship is likely to break down for a variety of factors. Perhaps this is because the nurse is unable or unwilling to see the patient as a person or judge whether professional power is misused or its influence unrecognised. This can also occur because the patient does not understand or accept his or her condition, hospitalisation or treatment. Another reason for asynchrony is if a person has either a physical or a psychiatric illness that makes communication very difficult. The challenges of both recognising and overcoming such barriers are an essential aspect of the skill of caring if we are to achieve and maintain effective partnerships with service users.

Morse went on to describe various strategies used by both nurses and patients to increase or decrease the level of the developing mutual relationships. In her study, nurses used activities that showed an overt demonstration of commitment by, for example, giving time, anticipating needs, getting to know the family and being the patient's advocate. On their part, the patients first of all assessed whether the nurse was 'good' in terms of displaying empathy and kindness, had a confident and gentle touch and was dependable (technical competency is assumed) and they then also used strategies by being what they saw as a 'good patient', being friendly and joking or trying to be 'no trouble'.

Morse found that if the nurse wanted to maintain control (thereby achieving a relationship based on inequality or asynchrony), they tended to depersonalise the patient, avoid eye contact, maintain an air of business and not be forthcoming with information, keeping patient and relatives 'in the dark'. On the other hand, some patients also used powerful tactics in trying to keep control by preventing the nurse from 'knowing' him or her, such as avoiding conversations which were of a personal nature, talking only of symptoms and treatment.

Morse's study is still pertinent today in emphasising that the nurse-patient interaction is an involved process in which both participants are 'giving' and 'receiving' and also that this is not a static process but ever changing. As in the Sukwinder story, some patients do not seem as if they want or need help initially but change as the relationship develops. It was 'commitment' that made Marjorie look for ways in which she felt she could help Sukwinder. Morse (199:467) also considered whether 'commitment' might be a more important and appropriate term to use than 'caring' in the nurse-patient relationship and preferred this as an alternative description. 'In the emotional sense, caring has notations of "fondness" or "love" neither of which may be present (or desirable) in a professional relationship.' However, perhaps rather than an alternative description, we would argue that commitment is yet another dimension of the caring process.

To think about

+ Think of a relationship with a patient/client in which you felt connectedness or mutual understanding. What were the factors that helped you to achieve this?
+ Think of a relationship with a patient/client that you felt was one-sided (there was asynchrony). What attempts were made or could have been made to overcome any negative consequences of this?
+ See if you can find parallels in your reflections with the Marjorie and Sukwinder story and/or with Morse's research study.

You might like to keep this information as part of your reflective learning diary, OAR or professional development portfolio.

Recognising the contributions of service users to a connected relationship

Memorable interactions may illustrate how service users may help nurses to look at things in a new light and influence their relationships. Thomson (2005: 71) wrote about one such event:

'I joined a team of nurses talking after the unexpected death of an alcoholic, homeless patient. They described how they had discovered a strong sense of fun in him when he taught some of them to dance. Their appreciation in him had increased his confidence, which in turn deepened their relationship with him – a magic moment.'

Through caring for others we gain many things. For example, Roach (2002) uses work by Mayeroff (1971: 30) to support this, suggesting that caring for others brings immense benefits to ourselves that we may not always recognise. 'By using powers like trust, understanding, courage, responsibility, devotion and honesty, I grow also; and am able to bring such powers into play because my interest is focused on the other.' Benner's (1984) important study of expert nurses also found that nurses benefited from what they did. They saw care as a two-way process and identified with their patients as active participants, not as passive observers.

This may involve an ability to respond in a sensitive way on the nurse's part. Look at the following incident described by Jamie, a student nurse, and think about how the community nurse responded to a patient's comment:

Case Study 2.2

'While out on my community placement with my mentor, I visited a man in his early sixties. Jim was an alcoholic and was practically bedridden, due to lying in bed all day and having a very bad diet. He smoked like a chimney – practically setting his bed alight with every cigarette. However, underneath the almost pathetic exterior, as well as a lonely and deeply sad man was an intelligent, gentle man. Jim's bed was by a window, overlooking the playground of a school.

As I stood up after finishing the dressing, which we were there for, I saw a tear fall down Jim's cheek as he stared at the children running happily below him. My heart went out to him and yet I could not find any words to say. Here was a man with no 'life' as I would call it, and yet this was the way he had chosen to live. I began to feel angry with my mentor. Why didn't she do something about the situation? Put him in touch with organisations to help, etc.? But deep down I knew as well as she did that this was the way Jim had chosen to live and we had no right to dictate our values to him.

As we were leaving, the tears still rolling down his cheeks, Jim said, with a touch of humour, "God, I'm a miserable old sod, aren't I?"

"Yes, Jim," said my district nurse, "but you can become very fond of miserable old sods sometimes, you know!" It seemed the perfect answer.'

Did you notice that this story began in the form of questions posed and answered by the student herself and ends with the magic moment of the humorous interaction between community nurse and patient, emphasising the connectedness of the relationship? The inclusion of Jamie's attention to detail in her story such as the 'tear rolling down his cheek' as Jim watched children playing in the playground (full of life as compared with him with 'no life') helps explain why her 'heart went out to him'. This shows the value of using detailed descriptions in your reflections. Jamie's attention to detail in her written reflection helps us to gain valuable insights into the patient's world. If we try to understand the story from her perspective, she is questioning whether people should 'be allowed' to live in a way that is risky and undesirable – an ethical dilemma. Her initial impulse was to say, 'Take Jim out of all this and make things better,' demonstrating how much she saw herself as a caring nurse. She reflected, however, on how she changed her mind and related this to the need to uphold personal choice (Jim therefore being 'allowed' to take an active rather than a passive role) and uncovering another way of valuing him and acknowledging his importance (another active role) by means of an appropriate humorous response from the community nurse. This 'caring' exchange, described as 'a perfect answer' denoting a positive, supportive and non-patronising attitude towards the patient, was an important opportunity of learning for Jamie. She recognised this through her reflection and this is likely to influence her practice in the future. This incident emphasises the importance of good role modelling. The student nurse recognised and valued the way the community nurse responded with skill and compassion. This kind of learning is emphasised by Firth-Cozens and Cornwell (2009), who note that role modelling compassionate care is a vital way of demonstrating its importance to younger staff and peers.

In spite of the less than ideal circumstances, the positive exchange between Jamie's mentor and Jim is likely to have contributed to a connected and mutual relationship. Jim could easily have been seen as an unequal partner in this relationship – his lifestyle was unhealthy and his behaviour could be seen as self-destructive. However, what was really apparent was that the nurse used the opportunity Jim provided in using wry humour to sum up how he felt about himself by responding in a similar manner – a warm and compassionate exchange from one human being to another. This is in line with Morse's description of a nurse–patient relationship that is built on reciprocity (a relationship in which one both gives to and receives from the other) and mutuality (a relationship based on shared trust and a feeling of affinity with the other).

Who is caring for whom?

From all this it follows that it may not be possible always to know who is benefiting most or even who is caring for whom. To illustrate this, Alex told of her experience as a patient in accident and emergency (A+E) after being knocked unconscious and suffering facial injuries following an unprovoked assault. Read her story and think about ways in which Alex was helping and supporting the student.

Case Study 2.3

'I was taken for a skull X-ray and a young student radiographer was left with me while the radiographers sorted out the equipment. After having several people around me all the time, I suddenly felt very lonely and when the student, trying to make conversation with me asked "How are you?" I burst into tears. The student looked very distressed and I realised that she must be feeling uncomfortable and probably didn't know what to say for the best. I didn't want her to feel like that so I tried to put her (and probably myself) more at ease by changing the subject. I said, "How long is your shift?" We chatted on about shift patterns for the few minutes which passed until the X-ray was ready to be taken.'

Many of these kinds of interactions occur all the time. You may have observed patients helping staff feel at ease (perhaps by initiating supportive conversations) and also patients sometimes do this with their relatives (perhaps trying to make them less worried by playing down unpleasant symptoms).

Another example of connectedness in the form of support, understanding and empathy is apparent in this next incident in which a nurse gave an account of her interaction with a family member. We think it is poignant in that, until a reflective workshop allowed her to explore the incident, the staff nurse who told the story overlooked the 'gift' she was given because she was distressed at her own perceptions of her inability to act in a supportive manner. When you look at the incident, think about significant features of the story in terms of how the newly qualified staff nurse was prepared for such an event and who helped her most.

Case Study 2.4

'A child had died on the early shift. I came onto the late shift with sister and a nursery nurse. I was a qualified nurse, but had no previous experience of a bereavement of a child. On the afternoon I was delegated to escort the child's grandparents to the Chapel of Rest to view their grandson. I was terrified and felt totally inadequate to cope with the grieving grandparents. I told sister this, but she informed me that I had to learn to cope with distressed relatives.

On walking to the Chapel of Rest I did not know what to say, so I kept quiet. On arrival I asked if they wanted to be alone, but grandmother insisted on me going in with her. I remember thinking to myself I have never seen a dead child before, and what will I do if the grandmother becomes hysterical? I felt totally useless and I must have looked it. I was taken by surprise when the grandmother took hold of my hand and said, "We will support each other, dear."'

You should notice that the nurse says that she had no previous experience of bereavement of a child. She says that she was terrified and felt totally unable to cope with the grieving grandparents. The sister's reaction that she had to learn to cope would not have diminished her feelings of fear and inadequacy. As an experienced nurse, the sister was in a position to reassure and advise, and perhaps you will think it should have been part of the staff nurse's preceptorship or induction programme, but it was the grandmother who took on the supportive role.

Why was the staff nurse 'terrified'? Perhaps she was reflecting her own fears related to the death of a child and felt that the relatives would be unable to cope and she would have to bear the responsibility of dealing with this. Despite her fears and perceived deficiencies in caring for the grieving grandparents, she still went with the grandparents to the Chapel of Rest, and kept quiet when not knowing what to say. We know that many of us are fearful of silence, eager to fill it with sound of some sort. However, words can be inadequate in some situations and silence can be a significant feature of 'connected' relationships, particularly if combined with appropriate touch. It should therefore be seen as an important part of the giving process.

In return for this staff nurse's courage, the grandmother gave her a wonderful gift when she took hold of her hand and said, 'We will support each other, dear.' Both the grandmother and Alex, in the previous story, were empowered by the support they gave. Instead of being 'victims' of the circumstances in which they found themselves, for a moment they became equal partners able to contribute to another's well-being. It is in the interest of professional health carers to appreciate this kind of mutual support and recognise the benefits gained.

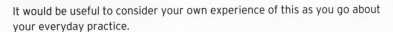

｛To think about

It would be useful to consider your own experience of this as you go about your everyday practice.

+ Identify and record examples of psychological support you have received from patients.
+ Reflect on whether you were able to acknowledge any reciprocal/mutual gifts of support.
+ When you have done this, consider whether this helps you to understand more the value of the emotional care you give to others.

You might like to keep this as part of your learning diary, OAR or professional development portfolio.

Learning further from our relationships

People who have learned to live with chronic conditions can teach us a great deal if we only listen! One nurse acknowledged the help she had from Jonah, a young man with paraplegia:

'A lesson I shall never forget is that Jonah taught me how to care for patients like him. He showed me how to prevent pressure sores. Early on in his hospitalisation, it happened to him and he didn't want it to happen to anyone else.'

The knowledge and experience of people with long-term conditions have been recognised as an untapped resource. In 2001, the Department of Health (DoH) published *The Expert Patient: A new approach to chronic disease management for the twenty-first century*. This emphasised the need to draw on the experience, knowledge and coping skills of people with long-term conditions such as heart disease, stroke, cancer, arthritis, diabetes mellitus, asthma, mental illness, epilepsy, and also help them towards self-management. An observation was made that health professionals often stated that 'my patient understands their disease better than I do' (DoH, 2001:4). The Care Quality Commission (CQC), the independent regulator of health and social care in England, went further, highlighting the importance of 'experts by experience' by involving them in monitoring the quality of care (see CQC annual report 2010/2011). Experts by experience are trained by various voluntary organisations and because their input has been particularly valued, there are plans to develop this further.

Most people with long-term conditions live in their own homes rather than in hospitals and this inevitably affects the kind of relationship they have with care providers. This will be explored in a later chapter but the focus on patients as experts through their experience has re-emphasised the importance of seeing each individual patient as a unique learning resource.

Learning from George

In spite of the emphasis in nursing education on the importance of work-based learning for personal and professional development, there is still a tendency to devalue and overlook how much can be learned from the most fundamental aspects of all care provision for every patient. This is illustrated by Ellie (a student nurse):

Case Study 2.5

'When I started my placement on the unit my mentor apologised for me being placed there, saying he was afraid it wasn't very "cutting edge". I am afraid that I also thought the same way because I had been so caught up with the advances in nursing and the technical skills that I had undervalued and had almost lost what I had once believed were important aspects of care.'

However, during Ellie's ward placement her reflections on her interactions with a patient led her to think again about why she had wanted to nurse in the first instance and also explore the current ideas she had about what it meant to care:

'Before starting my nurse training I believed that people wanted to be a nurse because they wanted to "care" about others. My first real experience of hospitals was through visiting my grandma who was admitted on a couple of occasions towards the end of her life. At every visit, on entering her side room there were things, I felt, that had been overlooked by staff. Her glasses would not be on or she would not have her teeth in; she had a hospital gown on when two of her own nightgowns were in the locker. On one occasion there was a plate of untouched sandwiches on the floor next to her chair and a cold cup of tea on the table over the bed, in which she had been left lying down. As she needed help with her mobility and was registered blind, I wondered how the staff thought she would manage to drink it. None of the nurses seemed to know anything about Grandma – they had just started their shift. These were not big things and the nurses, no doubt short-staffed, were busy with more important things. However, to a relative they conveyed a lack of care. "Who was looking after her?"'

When Ellie was in a practice placement during her first year as a student nurse, she had an experience that made her feel uneasy. She found that feeding a patient was not as easy as she had thought earlier. She began to realise that these 'small things/simple tasks/caring skills' are in reality quite complex, and offer opportunities for learning. As you are reading her account of her experience with George jot down what she might have learned from this experience.

Case Study 2.6

'I was on an early shift in a placement, working with people who were severely mentally impaired. I was asked to wheel a resident into the dining room and to give him his breakfast. This was not an unusual request. It was part of the normal morning routine, getting people up, washed, dressed and taken for breakfast.

But this was George. I had never fed him breakfast before or any other meal. In fact I hadn't really been involved before with any aspect of his care. There were a few other residents at the unit I hadn't had much involvement with just because that was how it had worked out. But I was conscious of feeling glad that I wasn't involved with George.

George dribbled constantly. I knew he couldn't help it, but he was always dribbling. He used to put his hands in his mouth and so always had saliva on his hands. When people fed him if they didn't look away from him he would just sit with his mouth open and not eat. If anyone caught his eye, be it staff or other residents, he would open his mouth and food would fall out. I hated saliva. Of all the bodily "fluidy mess" it was saliva I could not stand. And seeing people eat with their mouths open, seeing chewed-up bits of food in their mouths and on their hands, it could honestly make me gag.

As I pushed George along the corridor it was all I could think about. I wasn't going to be able to do it. I was going to feel repulsed by this poor man and it was going to be obvious. Going into the dining room a health-care assistant had just finished feeding one of the residents, I tried to catch her eye in the hope that she would send me off to get someone else up and feed George herself. But she didn't and I pushed George to the table. Someone in the kitchen put a bowl of cornflakes on the counter. "For George," they said. "Great!" I thought.

Milk seemed to pour out of his mouth and down his chin. I got up to get some paper roll to wipe it with. When I got back he had cornflakes all over his hands. I wiped them off and decided it would be best to wipe his mouth and hands after each spoonful. I got some more paper roll. We were halfway through the bowl before I realised that we were halfway through and I hadn't felt sick, I hadn't even pulled a face. He seemed a lot less messy than I thought.

Then I started to wonder if he was aware of not being able to control it and how much I would hate it if I were George. George leaned forward and put his hand on my knee, leaving a patch of gooey cornflakes behind. I looked at him, he smiled, and I smiled back. I thought, "It's nothing that won't wash off."'

Compare your findings with those of Ellie. When Ellie first started to reflect on the incident she wanted to focus on why the encounter had made such an impact on her. She was surprised and puzzled when she realised the experience she had with George was related to her thoughts about her grandmother's care and what she believed about good care (sadly opposite to what she had seen) and her reasons for choosing nursing as a career.

Reflecting on her experience had increased her self-awareness and prompted her to re-examine her core personal values. Jones's (2004) use of the psychodynamic notion of transference might have helped her to understand the complexities of nursing relationships. In this, patterns of relating to others are influenced by our experiences of past relationships. This can be positive (as in Ellie's case because it may have helped her to see George as a person, just as she had seen her grandmother when she was dependent on others, although it was a very different kind of relationship) but there is also the potential for relational difficulties if we project on to others negative feelings we have within ourselves. Ellie reflects in the next case study.

Case Study 2.7

'Through reflecting on the incident, I believe that I had projected my dislike of saliva on to George as a person. This helps explain why I had avoided contact with him. Whilst I was disappointed in myself for discovering this, in retrospect I was grateful the incident had occurred, as I was able to become more self-aware with regard to my feelings and subsequent behaviour.

Also, because of my nurse training, I knew that nursing skills involved procedures such as giving injections, setting up drips and carrying out observations such as blood pressures. My reflections helped me discover that I had started to consider that feeding a patient was not particularly a 'nursing skill' that had required a deal of expertise and knowledge. After all, I had assisted my grandma with her meals before undertaking any nurse training!

My feelings when involved with George were different from my feelings when caring for my grandma, and at first I therefore did not recognise this involvement as caring. I had found it easy to care for my grandma as I had an emotional bond with her. Caring for a stranger, I discovered, was not quite as easy.

One of my limitations was my aversion to saliva and I was put in a position that forced me to feed George. How I felt was incongruent with how I behaved, and I was conscious of the possibility that the inner self would betray the outer self. I feel I was eventually able to recognise I was caring for George because I fulfilled the task of feeding him. I paid attention to the little things, by wiping his mouth and hands during and after breakfast. I began to imagine how I would feel if I was in his situation and, by the end of the incident, I felt much empathy towards George.'

What else Ellie learned from the incident

Ellie found the incident helped her to consider many other aspects for which she needed literature to expand her knowledge and understanding:

'Looking at the literature on feeding I discovered that patients with dementia do experience feeding difficulties which change as the condition progresses These difficulties range from the refusal to eat, turning the head away, keeping the mouth closed, spitting out food, to leaving the mouth open and not swallowing. This links with George and with many other clients on the unit.'

This made her think again about the way in which she was feeding George and the type of food she was offering him. She also looked at a wider range of literature and other theories related to such topics as the psychosocial aspects of eating and drinking and of communication. She considered other concepts such as empathy and unpopularity and their relationship to the care she provided. The experience with George therefore contributed enormously to her learning and her future practice.

If we return to the incident, an important factor, which you may have noted, was the smile George gave to Ellie. This was an additional 'reward' for Ellie, influenced how she felt and helped to reinforce the importance of the learning she had gained about herself and what it was to truly care.

Whilst Ellie was searching the literature, she may have come across a similar kind of incident recounted by Redwood (2004:130), who was undertaking research into learning in practice. She observed a young nurse sitting by the bed of an elderly woman, trying to give her a drink of water. Just as in the incident with George described above, the nurse looked tense and anxious as the task was not easy and resulted in water constantly dribbling down the patient's chin and some choking and coughing.

'The nurse then repositioned herself and slightly moved the patient's head. This small adjustment made feeding the patient much easier. She then learned to go with the patient's rhythm of breathing through the mouth, sipping a little water, breathing through the nose and swallowing, followed by a moment's rest. Not too long to tire her patient, nor too short to rush her. I saw the nurse relax her body and develop an ease as she was slowly feeding her patient. She then began to speak slowly to the woman who responded by opening her eyes and looking at her. They spoke little, but for some time both women were in an intimate dialogue with each other.'

Once again, a task for someone had resulted in a key learning opportunity and a means of establishing 'connectedness'. For Redwood (2004:131) it was an opportunity for learning too which would influence her own development as a nurse researcher:

'I left the ward and I felt myself to be very fortunate. I realised that I had just witnessed a new member of our profession learn the highly complex and deeply human skill of enabling another person to drink. What I had seen was nursing. And I began to ask questions again. How did she learn the skill of feeding a patient who struggled to breathe? What happened between her and the woman that enabled her to learn from her?'

The above stories emphasise the importance of 'simple skills', which once unravelled do not seem to be 'simple' at all but complex and influential. They are at the essence of care and provide a vehicle for communication and learning. The student used the opportunity to learn about George by exploring her relationship with him and the skills and knowledge involved, focusing on these in her academic studies. There is an important lesson here for mentors in that similar opportunities will be occurring in practice on a daily basis but students may need guidance to recognise them. The influence of these interventions on the patient's care experience also needs to be taken into account when delegating to health-care support staff, whose contribution must be recognised, valued and supported, to ensure it is of high quality. Increased understanding of the importance of their role and the moves towards providing more formalised education and guidance for support staff will also help.

Time to think back

What has the incident with George taught us?

+ We have found that there is a great opportunity to provide sensitive and highly complex nursing care in areas which are often regarded as requiring little skill or expertise and to learn from the people for whom we care.
+ We can expand our ability to care by increasing our knowledge base, using theory to help explain and guide our practice.
+ Detailed and honest descriptive accounts of our experiences such as Ellie's can act as a springboard for immense learning.

Nurses have needs too

In discussing nursing, Bray (1998) is very forceful in her view that helping others is not an altruistic or unselfish act. As we have seen, nurses have needs in their relationships with patients and there are mutual benefits to be gained. Bray (1998:99) goes further to claim that we may be drawn to help others because of our own 'emotional wounds'. She points out the positive aspects of this. 'This is not necessarily a bad thing,' she suggests, since 'it makes good psychic and economic sense to heal oneself whilst promoting healing in others.' She goes on to quote Skynner (1989), who emphasised that mental health professionals 'are the only people willing and able to sustain their very difficult task of caring for others' mental illness perhaps precisely *because* they are getting something from it psychologically, something which they have been unable to obtain in the normal course of their life'.

We bring with us to every care situation emotional baggage or wounds, and for Kate, a student nurse, these may well have influenced the ways in which she cared for others with similar problems to her mother. She noted the time when she became more self-aware of her perceptions of her mother who had long-term mental health problems. Her written reflections on a visit to her mother in hospital recall the moment this occurred:

Case Study 2.8

'Everyone realises my mam is sick and there will never be a cure but it still gets me down at times. It's been happening since I was eight . . . The depression, the medication, the hospital etc. I can't remember the last time I was ever NOT worried about her.

I visited her the other day and she appeared a little better but not a lot. However, there was quite a weird moment between us that scared me to bits but I feel that it was meant to happen. I was sitting with her on her stiff hospital bed and whilst she was talking to me her voice seemed to settle into the background like an echo and I struggled to listen to her as I went back in time. She spiralled away from me and my mind began to burst with memories and thoughts of her when I was little - when I really looked up to her and wanted to be just like her. I adored the way she loved life and the people in it and how simultaneously everyone loved her back. I could picture her reassuring smile, warm eyes and the way she presented herself. She was a true lady and a perfect mother.

Suddenly my body overflowed with the sickening and abrupt sensation of shock with the mother I saw before me now. I couldn't make the link between when I was a child and that moment. I stared at her, wondering who she was and where she had gone . . . Lost within herself and saturated in drugs. I felt gutted and proud of her at the same time. Her soft voice with its depth of confusion flooded back to my senses and she was back on her bed next to me gripping my hands. All at once I realised that this too was my mother . . . I know that this will be probably seem abstract to you . . . I feel as though my inner self has grown and left the last skin of longing behind, like a butterfly. I feel free – free from grudges and bitterness, free from the past and free from my old disappointed searching self . . . '

Mental illness may affect our ability to see people as people, and the strength of Kate's story for us is that it highlights how easy it is to forget the individual even if it's someone close to us, and only see the condition or the difficulties surrounding them. It also demonstrates how beneficial it is when we remember them as human beings like ourselves with all our strengths and imperfections.

We need to recognise that nurses in all health-care settings gain potential benefits from acts of caring. We all carry with us learning behaviours influenced by previous experiences (positive as well as traumatic or hurtful) and so need to remind ourselves of the importance of developing self-awareness, perhaps by using reflection or by being able to engage in informal or formal support groups. In our working lives, we must recognise and accept that we all have needs, and are affected by our perceptions of how colleagues and patients interact with us. However, we need to be vigilant that we take care not to give less to those who seem to give less to us, such as those who might be categorised as 'unpopular' patients or clients.

Implications for informal carers

We can see that the act of caring for someone is complex and even in undertaking this for those we love, we are not doing so entirely for unselfish motives (the notion of altruism) since, as we have argued, the act of caring is not only beneficial for the recipient of the care but has important benefits for the care giver as well. Turner (2005) asks whether people ever act from altruistic or unselfish motives and the debate about whether altruistic behaviour exists has engaged academics such as philosophers, biologists and psychologists for a long time. This may seem a little abstract and remote for our everyday concerns but has practical and economic applications to health and social care.

To think about

+ Think back to what you have read about mutual benefits of care relationships. Does this have any relevance for informal carers?
+ What might make them go on providing care?
+ What might make them reluctant to continue?

Looking at research on this topic can help your considerations. Brouwer *et al.* (2005) found that almost half the informal care givers they studied (from a sample of 950 respondents) derived positive benefits from providing care themselves and that on average their happiness levels would decline if this care was handed over to someone else. This is an important point as it is so easy for people requiring care to see themselves only as a burden to others. Perhaps this indicates that there is a need for more acknowledgement of what care receivers are able to give to care relationships. The researchers also came to the conclusion that being in control of the process of caring seems to be particularly important for informal carers since once the 'caring starts to take control of them' (Brouwer *et al.*, 2005:97), the negative aspects outweigh the benefits. They therefore emphasised the need for assisting and supporting care givers to retain the benefits of providing informal care and retaining their sense of control over the situation. As we know, some carers labelled euphemistically as 'informal' may be providing care in very difficult and challenging situations (e.g. caring for a child who has complex care needs such as a tracheotomy, or a young woman with challenging behaviour, an older parent with Alzheimer's disease) and may need a great deal of support and help if they are to continue.

The research findings have relevance for us and need to be taken into consideration if we are to work effectively with patients and their families. We know that many families want to care for their loved ones at home, but we need to help them feel empowered to do this so that they are in control of the situation rather than overwhelmed by it. Carers UK is a charity that provides information for carers and campaigns on their behalf. On its website some of the difficulties faced by carers are discussed, including struggling to hold down a job, get a night's sleep, stay healthy and maintain relationships with friends and family. However, the view that caring can be a rich source of satisfaction in people's lives is also noted. 'It can strengthen relationships, teach a multitude of skills and help you to realise potential you never thought you had' (**www.carersuk.org**). Nurses can play a vital part in making carers feel valued and in helping them to overcome or minimise any difficulties encountered. In fact, creating and maintaining supportive relationships with informal carers are such an essential part of effective nursing care that we will revisit this important topic in more detail in Chapter 5.

Summary

In this chapter we have discovered, amongst other things, that:

+ Partnerships in nursing care can be very rewarding to both nurse and patient – it is a process of giving and receiving. Caring for others is connected with benefits to ourselves – one of mutuality and reciprocity.

+ There is a need to be aware of and accept emotional gifts from others. If we want to achieve true partnerships with patients we also have to acknowledge and value their contribution to our personal and professional growth.

+ Analysing our detailed reflections and using theory can help us gain more understanding of what it means to care,

+ It is important to help informal carers to maintain rewarding relationships with those for whom they care and we have to assist and support them so that they retain the benefits of providing care.

Looking forward

As you will see, we have collected additional caring indicators at the end of this chapter. These will be incorporated into our framework of caring at the end of the test. In the next chapter, in order to find out more about caring with compassion, we will use some stories that focus on inadequacies in care. It is these kinds of stories that are most often used to demonstrate that nurses are 'uncaring' and lack compassion. It is important to learn from these if we are to avoid difficulties and continue to develop caring and compassionate relationships.

Activity

+ When you next go into practice, pay particular attention to communica' that work well for both patient (and/or relatives) and you (or a colleague
+ It might be useful to make a detailed note of such exchanges so you can re   why a particular exchange was mutually beneficial.
+ Take note of the complexities of some skills in your area that might be considered as 'basic' or 'fundamental'.
+ Consider how your reflections can help you towards providing evidence for some of the outcomes and proficiencies you need for your professional development.

Caring indicators

1. Recognising what we give and what we receive in relation- ships
2. Demonstrating compassionate care through the ability to connect to or bond with others within the parameters of the professional role
3. Showing commitment demonstrated by giving time, identifying and acting on caring opportunities
4. Overcoming barriers in one-sided relationships, e.g. by seeing people as people, not as problems
5. Recognising the complexity and learning to be gained from 'simple' skills
6. Sensitivity and responsiveness to details and minute or covert signals
7. Demonstrating ability and openness to learn, through trust and honest exchange, from patients with experience and their carers
8. Assisting and supporting care givers to retain the benefits of providing informal care
9. Engaging in mutually beneficial communication exchanges, including the effective use of humour and silence
10. Recognising the importance of and utilising role modelling to demonstrate compassionate care

References

Barker, P and Davidson, B (1998) The heart of the ethical matter. In Barker, B and Davidson, B (eds) *Ethical Strife*. London: Edward Arnold.

Benner, P (1984) *From Novice to Expert: Excellence and power in clinical nursing practice*. Menlo Park CA: Addison-Wesley.

Bray, J (1998) Psychiatric nursing and the myth of altruism. In Barker, P and Davidson, B (eds) *Ethical Strife*. London: Edward Arnold.

Brouwer, W , Van Excel, N A J, Van den Berg, B, Van den Bos, G A M, Koopmanschap, M A (2005) Process utility from providing informal care: the benefit of caring. *Health Policy* 74, 85-99.

Care Quality Commission (2011) The state of health care and adult social care in England 2010-2011. London: The Stationery Office.

Carers UK *What is caring?* Available at: **www.carersuk.org** (last accessed 2/02/12).

Dignified Revolution. Available at: **www.dignifiedrevolution.org.uk** (last accessed 17/01/2012).

DoH (Department of Health) (2001) *The Expert Patient: A new approach to chronic disease management for the twenty-first century*. London: Stationery Office.

Department of Health (2008) *Confidence in caring; a framework for best practice*. London: Department of Health. Available at www. dh.gov.uk. (Last accessed 22/01/2012).

Firth-Cozens, J and Cornwell, J (2009) *The Point of Care; enabling compassionate care in acute hospital settings*. London: King's Fund.

Francis, R (2010) Independent Inquiry into care provided by Mid-Staffordshire NHS Foundation Trust January 2005-March 2009. London: Stationery Office.

Health Service Commissioner for England (2011) Report of the Health Ombudsman on 10 investigations into NHS care of older people. London: Stationery Office.

Jones, A C (2004) Transference, counter-transference and repetition: some implications for nursing practice. *Journal of Clinical Nursing* 14, 1177-1184.

Lindow, V (1996) What we want from community psychiatric nurses. In Read, J and Reynolds, J (eds) *Speaking our Minds: an anthology*. Basingstoke: Macmillan .

Morse, J M ((1991) Negotiating commitment and involvement in the nurse-patient relationship. *Journal of Advanced Nursing* 16, 455-468.

Redwood, S (2004) Case study 3: Careers in nursing research. In Freshwater, D and Bishop, V (eds) *Nursing Research in Context. Appreciation, application and professional development*. Basingstoke: Palgrave Macmillan.

Roach, M S (2002) *Caring, the Human Mode of Being* (2nd edn). Ottawa, Ontario: CHA Press.

Robertson, G (2010) Degree-only nursing: Are academic achievement and safe, compassionate care mutually exclusive? Panel debate available at **www.publicservice.co.uk/feature_story.asp?id=13581** (last accessed 22/01/ 2012)

Smith, P (2008) Compassion and smiles: what's the evidence? *Journal of Research in Nursing*, 13, 367-70.

Summers, S and Summers, H (2010) *Saving lives: why the media's portrayal of nurses puts us at risk*. New York: Kaplan Publishing.

Thomson, S (2005) Magic moments. *Nursing Standard* 19, 70-71.

Turner, D (2005) Altruism - is it still an anomaly? *Trends in Cognitive Sciences* 9, 317-318.

Chapter 3
Caring with compassion

LEARNING OBJECTIVES

By the end of this chapter you should have an understanding of:

1. What is meant by compassionate care and ways in which it is demonstrated
2. The importance of empathy and effective reassurance
3. The importance of attending to fundamental aspects of care to promote dignity and respect
4. The impact of small acts of kindness
5. The benefits and contributions that patients with experience make to our learning about compassionate care
6. The importance of raising concerns about poor professional practice

Introduction

In this chapter we will consider the impact of stressful or unhelpful interactions and interventions on service users and their families. Their stories will help us to consider situations in which nurses or other health-care professionals may not have been intentionally hurtful but nevertheless have caused tension, suspicion, distrust and distress. As nurses we need to face up to such situations and see what we can learn from them so that we will become more aware of such experiences and consider how we might deliver compassionate care by better promoting respect and dignity for the individual.

There have been strong debates in the UK concerning the need to improve fundamental patient care (Patients Association, 2011). Based on the four most frequent concerns that were received from patients, relatives and carers, the Patients' Association and the *Nursing Standard Journal* launched a joint campaign with the aim of promoting good nursing care. The complaints included patients not being helped to the toilet, nor given sufficient pain relief or sufficient nutritional intake and inadequate communication, e.g. call bells ignored. They set up the CARE Challenge asking nurses to use the following acronym to direct their care:

C – communicate with compassion
A – assist with toileting, ensuring dignity
R – relieve pain effectively
E – encourage adequate nutrition

It is easy to look for specific causes that have contributed to lack of attention to these most fundamental aspects of care, e.g. the nature of nurse education, lack of supervision or leadership, low staffing levels, inappropriate skill mix , increased bed/patient turnover, or heavy workloads, and all these need to be considered. However, based on the findings of a range of reports including Francis (2010) and the Health Service Commissioner (2011), it is the apparent lack of compassion which, it seems, is easier to identify when it is missing than when it is present, that has fuelled media outrage (Cornwell and Goodrich, 2008). It is important for us to consider how compassion is demonstrated, not only because it is at the heart of good nursing care but also because it has been found that the better relationships nursing staff can have with patients, the more confident patients will be with the care they receive (Department of Health, 2008).

What is compassionate care?

One of the difficulties in defining compassion is its subjectivity. 'Personal definitions fit in with our own view of the world, but may have little in common with the views of others.' (Davison and Williams (2009:16). Burnell (2009:319) also noted that compassion ' . . . is more than a professional mandate or attribute inherent in a care delivery model; it is characterized through actions that result when a nurse establishes a unique bond with a patient' (page 319). What is this unique bond? In many studies of compassion, it is linked with an understanding of another person's suffering (e.g. Nussbaum, 2001; Schantz, 2007; Younger, 2008). Van der Cingel (2011:680) also considers that sharing and understanding the effect of positive events are important for people with long-term conditions. 'When nurses see my distress and suffering, they also need to know about the events that keep me going and help me to survive, seems to be the argument.' Knowing more about patients as individuals in order to consider what actions will help them most is therefore another important requirement for showing compassion.

Van der Cingel's research in Holland also highlighted important differences between pity and compassion. In her study participants saw pity as having negative connotations. It can be pathetic and patronising, victimising the recipient and evoking feelings of powerlessness. 'This powerlessness "contaminates" the nurse as well,' states Van der Cingel (2011:683). 'As a result she is not able to support a patient any more.' She compared the Dutch word for 'pity' with the word for 'compassion', which she found had similarities in meaning for the participants in her research study but which had a much less negative connotation. Compassion exceeded the concept of simply sympathising with someone, but also involved a transfer of emotion likely to lead to helpful action. In her interesting and useful study, Van der Cingel (2011) concluded that compassion is valuable because it motivates patients as well as nurses and enables them to cooperate in achieving relevant outcomes of care. Thus compassion is seen as a vital component of good nursing care but its emotional aspects (perhaps what is meant by Burnell's 'unique bonding') need to be indicated through action. The terms 'empathy' and 'compassion' are sometimes used interchangeably and helpful action is a key component in Egan's (2001) definition of empathy. In the NMC's *Guidance for the care of older people* the part motivation plays in compassion is emphasised.

'You should also demonstrate compassion, which goes a stage further than empathy. Compassion is about not only having some feeling of what someone may be going through, but also caring enough to want to help and do something to make the situation better.' (NMC 2009:16)

Not waving but drowning

We have included incidents in this chapter that show lack of compassion and are traumatic and distressing because, unfortunate as they are, we need to face up to difficult situations and see ways in which we can take action to avoid such situations in the future and enhance our practice. User perspectives are particularly useful as a means of uncovering specific deficiencies in care that might be overlooked, thus helping us to increase skills in empathy and evaluate which interventions are helpful and which are not. Consider the following, written by Joanne, who reflected on her post-operative experience, and think about whether the nurse demonstrated compassion and helped her to feel safe.

Case Study 3.1

'I had a tracheotomy tube in and was not able to breathe properly. My mouth was swollen and I was gasping for air. I was trying to get the nurse's attention as she was at the foot of the bed, not looking at me. She was fiddling around with the charts, writing down my saturation levels.

I wrote "I can't breathe."

"Well," she said, "you are 100% saturated with oxygen."

I wrote "Yes, but I can't breathe."

This happened three times. I wanted an explanation, but she continued to stand at the bottom of the bed working on the sats. Then I noticed my husband, Dave, was there and he asked me, "What is the matter?"

I pointed at the nurse and made a fist. Here I was, three hours out of surgery and I wanted to bop somebody. Dave held on to my hand and said, "You're something else, you are!"

Because the nurse who had looked after me earlier had made me feel so good and cared for and calmed me, I was upset that the second didn't see my distress. It wound me up completely.'

To think about

+ Think about what we can learn from Joanne's story about reassurance as a positive way of demonstrating compassion.
+ Think about a situation in your own practice where you or someone else has given a patient or their relatives 'reassurance'. We need to understand exactly what we mean by this. Writing it down and reflecting (perhaps through the use of theory) will help to unpick the characteristics of effective reassurance. Read the next discussion to see how your findings match with ours.

You might like to keep this as part of your reflective learning diary or ongoing assessment record if you are a student. If you are a qualified nurse you could also use this as a topic to explore in your mentoring role.

Reassurance is a word that, as nurses, we often use but perhaps don't think enough about what it actually means. Teasdale (1995:79) saw it as 'an attempt to communicate with people who are anxious, worried or distressed with the intention of inducing them to predict that they are safe or safer than they presently believe or fear'. To do this we must first listen to someone, acknowledge their fears and take care not to respond in an overoptimistic or patronising way. Wynne-Jones (2006), who works as a GP, not only highlighted the importance of reassurance to reduce anxieties but interestingly she recognised other advantages of this in making her job easier in terms of reducing repeated questions and consultations. She suggested a communication framework consisting of five stages in the process of effective reassurance that you may find helpful:

+ eliciting ideas, concerns and expectations (she calls these ICEs)
+ checking and summarising these (this is a form of acknowledgement)

+ explaining what is happening and what can be achieved
+ checking understanding
+ entering into an agreement about a plan of action

In Joanne's case, the nurse appeared to listen but did not acknowledge her feelings. She looked for physiological evidence, significant as it was, but failed to take into account other important evidence – Joanne's fears and feelings. She therefore did not provide reassurance and evoke the calmness the first nurse had managed to obtain. She followed her own agenda, concentrating on the machine, and making Joanne feel that what she was saying was inconsequential. Joanne did not feel safe and therefore was not reassured.

A research study by Wilkin and Slevin (2004), on the meaning of caring in intensive care units, highlighted the significance of comforting as an important aspect of compassionate caring and, we would argue, reassurance. One of the participants described it as follows. 'Being comfortable is not just being pain free but being clean and feeling comfortable and not frightened of procedures, being reassured and relaxed and all this comes through good communication and psychological care' (page 53).

Literature provides support for the view that Joanne is not alone in this worrying kind of experience. Davies (2007) highlighted the significant number of intubated patients in intensive care units who have panic attacks and stressed the importance of constant reassurance by the nurse to minimise the symptoms. However, Wilkin and Slevin (2004:56), whilst acknowledging that technology has proliferated at a fast pace and potentially threatened the caring component of nursing, conclude that 'caring is not only possible within the technological world of ICU nursing but that it can be positively enhanced by nurses' mastery of the technological environment'. These authors stressed that this 'mastery' must involve utilising not only technical skills but seeing them as an opportunity to care in a holistic and empathetic way, described by one participant in their study as: 'It is about taking time and not getting too lost in all the entrapments of the machinery all around them' (page 54).

In the rush and bustle of a busy day at work it is all too easy to miss that first important step in reassurance and see people as objects to be processed rather than individuals and therefore miss, ignore or misinterpret the signals of distress. In the interaction described above, Joanne's feelings of being misunderstood and her unrecognised anxiety remind us of a poem by Stevie Smith (1981:131), reproduced with permission, entitled 'Not Waving But Drowning', which begins:

> *Nobody heard him, the dead man,*
> *But still he lay moaning:*
> *I was much further out than you thought*
> *And not waving but drowning.*

Joanne thought she was 'drowning' and the nurse did not allay that fear. She was able to contrast this with the previous care she had received where her perception appeared not to be based on the nurse's use of higher technical skills, but, rather, on a caring and empathetic approach that she valued.

The need for reassurance is also important for those needing acute and crisis mental health interventions. A report from MIND, the mental health charity in the UK, indicated the importance service users placed on the quality of the human interaction involved. (MIND 2012). They reported that they wanted to be respected and taken seriously, experience warm, caring, and compassionate responses and be shown understanding. The Inquiry panel concluded that such attitudes can be life saving and provide a basis for recovery. One participant explained this as follows:

> 'I needed a safe place – somewhere where I could not seriously harm myself until I recovered emotionally. I also needed to feel that someone actually cared about me so that I would not leave hospital in the state of mind where I still wanted to harm myself because I felt that no one cared about me.' (page 13)

The evidence indicates that reassurance can have wide-reaching effects and be undertaken in a number of ways since physical and emotional aspects are interrelated both in cause and effect. Williams and Irurita (2006:408) studied perceptions of hospitalised patients in Australia and found that emotional discomfort was identified 'by the experience of unpleasant feelings such as fear, frustration, sadness, worry, anger, stress, anxiety, tension, embarrassment, pessimism about life, low spirits, helplessness, and despondency'. However, the conditions that caused emotional discomfort could be physical, such as the experience of unpleasant physical sensations like pain, tiredness, dizziness, weakness, shortness of breath, restricted movements, skin irritations, hunger, and feeling cold. It would seem that therapeutic reassurance in its deepest sense does not mean just superficial niceness but a requirement by the nurse to develop all her skills in empathy, nursing observations and interventions and also in managing the environment in which care is provided.

Empathy as an indicator of compassionate care

Empathy is often defined as the ability to put oneself in another person's shoes and is described by Rogers (1991) as the basic requirement for 'seeing' and 'hearing' in client-centred approaches. However, Skidmore (2005) also points out the uniqueness of every experience and he refers to Buber (1958), who argues that at best we can only gain a perception of someone else's experience. He suggests that we share 'affective resonance' but not the shared history, so every experience of emotional pain/trauma is unique to that person. It would appear that for Joanne the first nurse who cared for her had developed 'affective resonance' but the second had not.

Sometimes our deficiencies are inadvertent rather than deliberately cruel or unsympathetic, but only by reflecting on examples of situations will we become aware of what people have found distressing and so will we be able to have greater insight into our own behaviour and the impact we might have on others. Developing empathy is therefore an ongoing learning process but being aware of it will have a direct relationship on the plan of action we take and the care we provide. Chambers and Ryder (2009:33) put empathy into practical terms for nurses by noting 'If we can glimpse the "private world" of our patients, in all its distress, whilst keeping the "as if" quality, we can empathise with them, without feeling submerged and unable to help them.'

It may be seemingly minor incidents that have a great significance for participants and require empathetic exchanges. Esther described how anxious she was visiting her husband, who had just been admitted to a trauma unit following a road accident. She approached a staff nurse who was standing at a notes trolley to ask how her husband was and what was likely to happen next. The staff nurse did not look up from the trolley but continued to look through the notes, saying 'He's OK - we'll know more when the doctors do their round tomorrow.'

Although this incident might seem insignificant and the response adequate, the lack of the small act of looking up and maintaining eye contact meant that Esther came away with the perception that the staff nurse was uncaring and did not realise the importance of the information she had been asked to give. The small act of looking up, maintaining eye contact and looking interested would have made all the difference to Esther, who left with suspicions about the quality of care that was likely to be provided for her husband. The inference can be drawn that the nurse thought she was too busy with more important work but in actual fact changing her behaviour in such a small way would not have taken any more time. Findings related to the predominance of a 'task-orientated' approach to communication were also found in a study of patients' perceptions of nurse communication (McCabe, 2004).Unfortunately, according to the author this approach resulted in patients feeling that the tasks were more important than they were and consequently they did not like to bother the 'busy nurse'.

Goffman's (1969) studies of 'roles' we play in life emphasised the influence of context and perception. In the case of Esther, described above, she seems almost a 'non-person' – her perceived role not important enough to engage in significant interaction. Buber (1958), an influential philosopher, has written about different ways we relate to others, which may help us to understand Esther's perception. He talks about 'I-Thou' and 'I-It' relationships. It is only when we truly relate to another that we enter into an 'I-Thou' relationship; everything else he considers can be regarded as 'I-It' relationships – we regard others as we would objects.

We can draw parallels for this in the staff nurse's exchange with Esther and perhaps in the findings of task-orientated communication with patients. Without providing eye contact, warmth or interest, Esther's exchange with the staff nurse became an 'I-it' encounter rather than an 'I-Thou'. It is important to remember that even brief exchanges like this can have an enormous influence on the way service users and their families perceive the care received, particularly the confidence they have in that care (Department of Health, 2008).

Personal evaluations of services are particularly significant if care is to be more personalised and responsive (Department of Health, 2007, 2008). Esther said her experience made her feel 'invisible' and powerless and many others have reported feeling this way, particularly older people (Department of Health, 2006). Acknowledgement of the individual can therefore be seen as a good indicator of compassionate care. Conversely, it is all too easy for nurses to engage in 'distancing' techniques (see Chapter 4) in order to protect themselves and their time (particularly when extremely busy or short-staffed), but in doing so dignity and respect, for those being cared for, can be compromised.

Time to think back

Empathy is an important concept and you might want to think back on your own personal experiences where you felt that someone had become very close to understanding and entering 'your world' and because of this was able to help you in some way. You could also contrast this with an experience where you were not able to convey your needs and felt like a 'non-person' even if it was for a brief period of time. Understanding your own reactions to situations will help you empathise with others.

Dignity and respect

The importance of recognising needs and maintaining dignity and respect for older people was highlighted in the Philip Report undertaken for the Department of Health (2006), *A new ambition for old age: Next Steps in Implementing the National Service Frameworks for Older*

People. The report referred to the number of high-profile cases of poor treatment in mental health and general hospitals, in care homes and domiciliary care. 'Our definition of dignity is based on the moral requirement to respect all human beings, irrespective of any condition they may suffer from' (Department of Health, 2006:4). The appointment of key nurses was proposed to ensure that older patients are treated with dignity and respect. In addition a Dignity Code was launched by the National Pensioners Convention in February 2012 aimed at upholding the rights and maintaining the dignity of older people (**www.ncpuk.org**) throughout all care services.

Whilst we would argue that these are important strategies to protect the interests of vulnerable people, we see them as an indicator of failure - that the importance, value and impact of caring approaches have not been understood, measured or given enough attention in everyday practice whether in hospital or community care situations. It seems it is often only when caring is missing at such a high level that it is noticed by the public and the press that it becomes the focus for discussion and action, but it is what nursing is all about.

Consider the following story told by Miriam and jot down all the inadequacies in the care provided.

Case Study 3.2

'My mum had a stroke two years ago but after a while, because she's so independent, she managed to continue living on her own with the family popping in regularly to help her out when she needed it. Unfortunately not long ago she had a lingering chest infection and when she developed chest pain, she was admitted to hospital. She's in her eighties so we were really worried about her as she seemed so frail. We were really upset to see her getting weaker very quickly and the lady in the next bed said that she wasn't eating at all but her meals were often taken away as nobody came to help her. She herself had mentioned it to the nurses and one came to help with the next meal but since then they seemed to have forgotten that she needed help.

I was also upset to find that my mother was now incontinent and one day she started to cry and told me that the night nurses had told her off for wetting the bed. I didn't know what to do for the best but at least I thought I could make sure she was fed so I asked permission to come in at mealtimes and help my mum and the sister said this would be very helpful as they were so short-staffed.

One morning I was helping Mum with her breakfast. As I sat feeding her, Mrs Jones (in the bed opposite) rang the buzzer and asked to go to the toilet. The nursing assistant said, "Can't you wait till after breakfast, Betty?" Mrs Jones said she was desperate so the nurse went for help and two of them, rather crossly, got her out of the bed and took her on a chair to the toilet. They hadn't covered her up properly and so her bottom was on full view to the rest of the room.

Later I overheard the two nursing assistants washing another old lady (behind the screens). What really horrified me was that it was obvious they were not talking to the patient but were discussing in great detail their escapades from their night out. I was embarrassed - and I consider myself broad-minded! Their discussions shocked me. So much for care - I was really glad to take my mother home.'

Compare your findings with ours

We found that there were many faults in the care provided, such as there was not enough assistance from staff to ensure Miriam's mother's nutritional needs were met. This reflects findings by Age Concern (2006:4) that 'One of the most frequent issues raised with Age Concern by the relatives of older people who have been in hospital is the lack of appropriate food and absence of help with eating and drinking for people who are unable to manage this for themselves.' Their campaign, 'Hungry to be Heard', set out seven steps to reduce the risk of malnourishment of older people when in hospital (you can find these by accessing the Age Concern website at **www.ageconcern.org.uk/**). Unfortunately, various reports in the UK – the Francis report (2010), the CQC State of Care Report (2011) and that by the Health Service Commissioner for England (2011) into NHS care of older people – underlined the need for continued vigilance and action to alleviate this.

Being told off for wetting the bed would have made Miriam's mother embarrassed and feel that she was regarded rather like a naughty child. This would make her feel undignified, would have affected her self-esteem and showed a complete lack of respect and acknowledgement of her needs. Her incontinence could be a result of a general lack of care and attention. The way staff regarded toileting needs as an 'inconvenience' could also be seen in the way they responded to Mrs Jones's request. This was an uncaring approach and showed a lack of the empathy that's so necessary for compassionate care. In other words, staff were not meeting what Noddings (2003) describes as the 'ethical demands' of caring.

Miriam might have found it difficult to complain about the service because of concern about how the staff might see her as a troublemaker and she might have thought a complaint could affect the care provided for her mother. The Patient Advice and Liaison Service (PALS) exists to help people like her. This service was created to provide on-the-spot help in every NHS Trust by listening to patients' and families' concerns, identifying gaps in services and acting as a catalyst for change. In Miriam's case, PALS could also have given advice about the local complaints procedure. The NHS Constitution (Department of Health, 2012) emphasises the rights of service users and their families (and staff) to voice and receive feedback if they have any concerns about the quality of care received without fear of adverse effects. (See NHS Choices (**www.nhs org.uk**) for detailed information about the NHS complaints procedure.) However, it is likely that even with formal and more open and accessible procedures in place, some service users will still be reluctant to do so. There is a need therefore to look at ways in which concerns can be voiced before they cause major emotional distress and physical problems. Early studies on 'intentional rounding', in which health-care staff make regular checks on individual patients at set times, have shown increases in patient satisfaction (Bartlett, 2011).

Staff called Mrs Jones 'Betty'. They would have needed to ensure that this was the name that she wished to be called by, otherwise they could be being overfamiliar and treating her again with disrespect. In addition, Mrs Jones was taken to the toilet inadequately covered. This showed disrespect and lack of understanding of Mrs Jones's needs for privacy and dignity. It would also have affected the way other patients in the ward thought they were regarded.

Staff were ignoring a patient whilst giving her intimate care (an example of 'I-It' rather than 'I-Thou'). Their focus was on themselves and their own preoccupations rather than the person receiving the care. It was also insulting to both the individual and all the other people in the room as they were overhearing inappropriate and embarrassing comments. This was truly uncaring care.

It is our contention that there is a need to become aware of situations such as Miriam has provided and to look at ways in which we can improve care for all patients, to ensure we do not engage in discriminatory practice, particularly towards those who are vulnerable such as children, older people, those in long-term care and those with learning disabilities or mental health problems. It should also be remembered that one of the most important ways of conveying respect and therefore promoting dignity is through effective and sensitive communication (Price, 2004).

The Dignity in Care campaign was set up in response to public concern in the UK about the loss of dignity for older people in care (see **www.dignityincare.org.uk**). Their 10-point Dignity Challenge depicts what high-quality services that respect people's dignity should include:

1. Have a zero tolerance of all forms of abuse.
2. Support people with the same respect you would want for yourself or a member of your family.
3. Treat each person as an individual by offering a personalised service.
4. Enable people to maintain the maximum possible level of independence, choice and control.
5. Listen and support people to express their needs and wants.
6. Respect people's right to privacy.
7. Ensure people feel able to complain without fear of retribution.
8. Engage with family members and carers as care partners.
9. Assist people to maintain confidence and a positive self-esteem.
10. Act to alleviate people's loneliness and isolation.

It is not surprising that staff can feel that they are having an uphill battle to provide good-quality care and we can look to many reasons why this is not occurring. It could be related to extremely heavy and demanding workloads, inappropriate staff or skill-mix levels, weak leadership or inadequate training or supervision, but we also have to recognise that some individuals may not be meeting professional standards and expectations.

Whistle blowing as part of compassionate care

There is a history of difficulties undergone by nurses and other health and social care staff after they have aised concerns about poor standards of care. In 1990, Graham Pink, a nurse, brought to light inadequacies in the care of older people in Stepping Hill Hospital in numerous letters written to the hospital management and members of parliament, until he finally went public in the press. He was dismissed in 1991 for breaching confidentiality. When he appealed, the case was settled before an industrial tribunal reached a verdict. There have been a number of 'high-profile' cases since that time but the inquiry into the care provided by Mid-Staffordshire NHS Foundation Trust (Francis, 2010) brought wide public attention to the need to give more clarity for staff re the raising of concerns and clearer whistle-blowing policies and safeguarding procedures. At the time of writing, there has been a pledge to make further changes to the NHS Constitution reflecting the expectation that staff should raise concerns at the earliest opportunity and be supported without suffering any detriment.

The NMC Code: *Standards of conduct, performance and ethics for nurses and midwives* (2008:4) stipulates that 'speaking up on behalf of people in your care and clients is an everyday part of your role, and just as raising genuine concerns represents good practice, "doing nothing" and failing to report concerns is unacceptable'. It sets out how a nurse should do this:

> *2.1 you must act without delay if you believe that you, a colleague or anyone else may be putting someone at risk*
> *2.2 you must inform someone in authority if you experience problems that prevent you working within this code or other nationally agreed standards*
> *2.3 you must report your concerns in writing if problems in the environment of care are putting people at risk*
> *2.4 as a professional, you are personally accountable for actions and omissions in your practice, and must always be able to justify your decisions.*

A whistle-blowing helpline for NHS staff (extended to staff and employers in the social care sector) was set up in 2112 (**www.nhs.org.uk**).

Forgetting to ask what is needed

One way in which we can eliminate the possibility of poor care is by working in closer partnership with patients and their families. As we have seen, attention, to both the artistry and the science of care, is necessary to give effective holistic care. We may be so engrossed in the tasks that are evident that we may simply forget to ask what is needed. A similar experience to Miriam's was identified by West (2006:29), a nursing student who, as a result of her experience when visiting a friend (a patient in her seventies), realised the importance of proactive care.

> 'She was so quiet and unlikely to ask for help that I was worried that she had just been left. She was in pain but would not ask for relief – how could she when she was unable to see the call button? She was thirsty, but no one had thought to pour her a drink and place it within her reach . . . The ward nurses were not bad nurses – they were happy to help whenever I asked, but was this enough?'

It may well be quiet and compliant patients who do not gain the care they need because we are not assessing them adequately. Proactive interventions are an essential part of the caring process and these may be the result of assessment based on overt cues (signs of distress, dehydration, breathlessness, etc.) as well as a result of asking the patient and/or their relatives what they need. In the rush and bustle of ward routines and procedures and even in a limited amount of time available to make a community visit, something obvious can easily be missed or assumptions can be made. As mentioned earlier in this chapter, intentional rounding, where service users are asked if they have any concerns or needs, rather than waiting for them to initiate this, may help overcome this problem.

Consider the next scenario, which highlights the importance of recognising the dangers of making assumptions and drawing inappropriate conclusions, sometimes transferred to others within a handover report.

Case Study 3.3

'The parents of a nine-month-old baby, who had been receiving chemotherapy on the ward, had just been told that he was not responding to treatment and nothing more could be done for him. They were given the option of staying in hospital or taking him home to die. The parents decided they would stay in hospital. I was on the late shift the day that this news was given to them and at the handover we were told that the family needed time to just be together and to keep nursing intervention to a minimum.

I felt worried about going into the room to give the baby his medication in case I upset the family. On entering the room, I was greeted as warmly as I always had been. The mother asked what was wrong as they had hardly seen anyone. I explained that the staff felt that they needed some privacy without nurses interrupting. This, I discovered, was not at all what they wanted and they felt abandoned by staff. They had elected to stay in hospital as they valued the support they had been given and wanted to continue as they felt it would make it easier for them to cope.

On reflection, I realised that the decision to give them privacy had been an assumption by my colleagues as to what the family wanted. I also wondered if it was a way of all of us being able to avoid a painful experience for ourselves. Put in a similar situation again, I realised I should try to negotiate what families really want, rather than try to assume their needs.'

You will have noticed from the above that the nurse recognised that she and other members of staff might have been avoiding the family almost unconsciously to lessen the distress they too were experiencing. We all do this and may resort to unconscious avoidance measures and overlook personal needs.

Other factors may influence our tendency to make assumptions. Claire told us of her experience when Penny, her 10-year-old daughter with severe learning disabilities, went into hospital. Penny uses sign language to communicate. It is not Makaton, but her own modified version because she has poor 'fine motor movements' so is unable to use her fingertips appropriately.

Case Study 3.4

'You have to really know Penny to be able to read what she is signing. She also conveys a lot with her facial expressions and eye movements. To someone else these are easily missed because they are so subtle. If we are not with her, she cannot communicate. When she went into hospital, she was signing "drink" and the nurses did not understand. Fortunately we were there, so we knew. There are other things - all of her food and drink has to be tepid, otherwise she will spit it out, looking as if we are trying to poison her. Without knowing her, the individual cannot care for her. Her right arm has to go in first when we are dressing her - this really matters to her. If one thing is not quite right, she refuses to do anything! Imagine not being able to tell people what you need, like the basics for life itself.'

To think about

+ Think of a practice situation in which you believe you have anticipated someone's needs and consider what evidence you used to come to that conclusion. Did you:
  - follow a care plan?
  - follow a role model?
  - base your intervention on previous experience?
  - look for verbal and non-verbal cues from the patient, relatives?
  - use observational charts?
+ You will have learned many ways to assess patients' needs, all of which are important and add to the overall picture. Has this chapter made you think again about the importance of asking the patient or their relatives how they view their needs?
+ Consider whether we are always able to meet these expressed needs or whether we have to sometimes use other strategies such as realistic but empathetic negotiation.

You might like to keep this as part of your reflective learning diary or ongoing assessment record.

Using patient experience

Listening to stories from patients and their relatives helps us to understand their lived experience and therefore recognise ways we might help. Warne and McAndrew (2005) stress that seeing patients as experts in their personal and cultural background and in the story of their illness can help maintain identity and lead to an exchange of important information and knowledge on the part of both patient and nurse. Each has an important part to play in this. 'Patient experience knowledge is different from the knowledge that is gained in grounding theoretical knowledge or practice knowledge – but it is part of both . . . Patient experience knowledge requires the nurse to move their gaze from the body (as an object of intervention) to the person living a life' (Warne and McAndrew, 2005:17). This way, they claim, nurses may better understand non-cooperative behaviour, non-compliance and the meaning interventions have for the patients. This is another example of the importance of the I-Thou relationship.

Angelica had had a number of radical operations and extensive radiotherapy after she was found to have adenocarcinoma of her tongue base. The surgical procedures involved removal of a significant part of her mouth, tongue, salivary glands and the nodes around her neck. Also, because she had to have her tongue removed, she was given an operation that took part of her muscle from her lower shoulder to make her a new tongue. Angelica had speech therapy and had to learn to eat again. Her account of her everyday life helps us to see her as an individual – a young woman still trying to lead as normal a life as possible but whose needs have changed dramatically. Think about how the nurses might have met Angelica's need to communicate.

Case Study 3.5

'The social side of my life, the quality of life I have now has changed . . . I can't even have a normal meal with my friends because of my having to have peg feeds . . . And, because I can't speak properly, some people act as if they think that there is something wrong with me mentally. But I do go out and join in. I eat the soup, although it takes me forever. For instance, recently my friends and I were having a meal in a restaurant and we were having a good time. I had a mouthful of soup. There was something funny I wanted to say but, because it takes me ages to even eat soup, it was about five minutes before I managed to swallow it. When I had my mouth empty the moment was gone for my punchline - it was not funny any more.

   The same kind of thing had happened to me in hospital. The nurses always seemed too busy and I was often desperate to tell them something important but it took so long to get it out that often the moment was lost.'

Finding time

We think Angelica's story stresses that even if we're very busy it is important to find time to give patients the opportunity to communicate and therefore we need to find ways of enabling them to make their feelings and needs known. Parker (1999) highlights the problems of intubated patients in intensive care units who, like Angelica, experienced distress related to their inability to release emotional tension and gain comfort through conversation. Her study also indicated that they were often not consulted about their care and they 'felt as though they were alone in a world removed from the world of others' (Parker, 1999:65). Not only is empathetic communication beneficial in terms of showing kindness and concern but it may well ensure that less time is needed in future to calm distressed patients. Parker (1999) described how frightened patients would sometimes panic and react violently by pulling out tubes, lashing out or trying to get out of bed.

   If we are proactive, looking ahead rather than reacting to situations as they occur, patients will feel that we respect them and want to help. In Parker's study, patients most often remembered staff with particular characteristics - those who were competent, kind, showed empathy and conscientiousness. Making sure that people do not feel neglected, even in hectic periods, is important and many nurses do this by renegotiating when they will be able to spend time with them. It is often these small actions that make people feel they are not forgotten.

Simple acts of kindness

Stories from patients also help illustrate the importance of simple acts of kindness as Georgina described.

Case Study 3.6

'I had just come back from the operating theatre [after a facial operation] and the nurse was lovely. Everything was hazy, probably because of the morphine. I am not sure of the time but I don't think I had been back very long from the operating theatre. I sent my husband home. The nurse told me my mother rang. It was lovely to be contacted. The nurse washed

me down and made me clean. I was intubated and ventilated so there was no way of communicating at the time except in writing.

   She said, "I am going to get a mirror." I had the option to look. I could have said no. But I
did and that was good. This got it into my head that I hadn't changed that much. I think it was
being touched that made me feel human and accepted. That was a calming period and I slept.'

For patients such as Georgina, the need to maintain one's identity is particularly important and as professionals we may forget what aspects may have an impact on this, such
as: being touched and reassured in small ways, being kept clean, being involved in small
decisions, receiving information such as calls from family and the reassurance of a recognis-
able self-image. This is reinforced by Magyar, who gave this account of how she felt about a
change to her appearance.

Case Study 3.7

'I had gone into hospital for one operation that should have taken me about one week to
recover but I was in for four weeks. Before I was admitted I had planned to let my hair cover
the scar on my neck so that it would not be so noticeable. They put about four or five elastic
bands in my hair to tie it up before I went to theatre and my hair was put up into a paper
hat. I had a bandage around my neck and tied at the top of my head. Like in the cartoons.
Eventually they took the bandage off and I had dried blood in my hair but I was pleased as I
now thought I could wash my hair once I got home.

   'But my curly hair had grown around the elastic bands. Peter tried all one afternoon (at
home) but couldn't manage. So, then the hairdresser tried, for example with olive oil. I was
there in the hairdresser's all day with my nasogastric tube and they tried very hard to give
me some privacy. They finally had to cut my hair off. This broke my heart. I was inconsolable.
Peter said, "I can't believe you would cry over this. Everything you have gone through . . . the
operation - you never complained, you never cried. And they cut your hair off and . . . " '

We also saw an example of this in Chapter 1, with Alan Bennett's description of the effect
of his mother's hair being washed and left uncombed and uncurled after admission to hospital, so that it 'stood round her head in a mad halo' making it difficult for him to see how
she would ever return to her 'normal' self. For Magyar the cutting of her hair had a similar
devastating effect. Perhaps had the nurses known about the effect of the bands they would
have thought of another strategy.

   Acts of unkindness or insensitivity can lead to non-compliance in treatment. You can see
how this happened in Lauren's story.

Case Study 3.8

'Postoperatively, I had many complications including breathlessness and I needed oxygen
for this. It was decided that I would need to use the C Pap machine. Instead of this being
explained to me and introduced to me gradually, the mask was forced on to me, with

someone sitting on my hands! Perhaps it is not surprising that I panicked and refused to have this on. I was very upset. I wanted to go home. The female doctor declared that I would not even make it to the door and told me that if I refused to have the machine on then she would intubate and I would be awake. I did feel that I could have been treated in a kindlier manner by the nursing staff and the female doctor.

Following this I was visited by a male doctor who explained how the C Pap machine worked and why I needed it. As a result of this I agreed to try again and I managed to keep the machine on as long as I could put it on myself and I knew it would be removed if I panicked.'

Relating to and working with Lauren instead of using a confrontational approach changed a difficult situation into a collaborative partnership with a more effective outcome for all. Many patients remember other small acts of kindness that have had great significance for them, including Sharon.

'There were two excellent nursing staff on the night shifts. They washed my hair, they laughed with me, and they were friendly and reassured me that they would not leave me when they realised I was terrified. But I cannot remember their names – however, I do know that I prayed every evening for these two to be on duty.'

The outcomes of simple acts of kindness are often hidden. The staff nurses referred to by Sharon may not have been aware of the therapeutic effect of their interactions. Sometimes somewhat casual interactions can produce quite dramatic changes, and health-care professionals who are sensitively attuned can change a difficult encounter into a more congenial one. A student nurse wrote of his experiences in A+E department.

Case Study 3.9

'One afternoon a qualified nurse ran up the ward to ask for help with Mick, a patient. He was quite well known to us since many of the staff had experienced episodes of violence with him, so we all went immediately. Mick was standing in the side room swearing like a trooper. We all tried to calm him down but this did not work. His language got worse as he got more agitated and I found this the hardest part. If anyone I knew called me these names I would have walked away from them – but here I had to stay and try to help calm him down.

Bill, one of the health-care assistants, remarked wryly, 'This is just like being at a Sunderland versus Newcastle game.' With that, Mick stopped and looked at Bill.

"Do you support Newcastle, Mick?" Bill asked.

Mick replied, 'F–No! I don't watch rubbish. I support a proper team.'

It was the breakthrough we had all been waiting for. A conversation about football ensued and helped defuse a difficult situation.'

The student identified how an almost 'throwaway' remark provided the stepping-off point for perceiving Mick as an individual with his own place and preferences in society rather than 'the violent man with a psychiatric history'.

To think about

+ Think about any proactive interventions you made last time you were on duty and how these will have affected the quality of the care you provided.

You might like to keep this information as part of your reflective learning diary or as evidence for your ongoing assessment record or portfolio. These aspects could be a useful topic for discussion during mentorship or supervision.

The effects of not paying attention

As we have said, we are not advocating a truly caring approach for humanistic reasons alone, important though these may be. If unthinking and ritualistic practices are followed, dire consequences may occur. Liam illustrates what can happen if something unexpected is not recognised and therefore not taken seriously:

Case Study 3.10

'I began to feel extremely hot every afternoon. I needed a fan and I kept saying, "I don't feel very well", "Do you think it is an infection?", "Do you think that is pus around the drain? It looks green to me". One senior staff nurse kept telling me over and over again that it was just oozing lymphatic fluid. My temperature, she said, was normal. But they only took it once a day on a morning. But I felt more and more ill – I felt faint and kept feeling as if I was passing out. I was too tired to protest further. My mother told me later that when she got home from visiting me she got on her knees and prayed, she was so worried about me. By the end of that week my mother, my partner and others could not believe how ill I was and were very worried because they did not have faith in what they were being told. They got together and managed to get the consultant in to look at me on the Saturday. I then got intravenous antibiotics and they removed the drains. The pus spurted out from the hole every time they dressed the wound. It was a severe infection.'

Liam who told us this story never wanted to go back to that particular hospital again; although other people will have different experiences, nothing could erase the fear and anguish he had in being disregarded. In some ways he was fortunate in that he had family and friends who were his advocates and played an important role in getting the care he required.

Partnerships in care – who knows best?

We must recognise that family and friends may find it difficult to get through the covert or hidden power that professionals and organisations hold and there may be problems in how they all work together to make decisions about the best care for the patient. Carol, a student nurse, expressed her concern about how staff, believing that they were doing the 'right' thing for the patient, deceived a relative who had a different view.

Case Study 3.11

'Fred is 70 years old and has suffered many strokes in his lifetime that have left him completely immobile, mute and a victim of dementia. He is also blind. Joan, Fred's wife, lives in the home she shared with her husband before it became too difficult for her to care for him on her own. She comes to visit Fred once a day, having either lunch or tea with him. Joan has frequently expressed her wish to be involved in all aspects of Fred's care. She believes that in knowing him better than anyone else she is capable of standing in as his voice . . . A speech therapist visited Fred and expressed concern that one day he might choke. She advised that all of his meals were to be liquidised in order to reduce this risk. All staff agreed with this; however, Joan did not.

After listening to the speech therapist and almost every staff member explaining why it was a good idea, Joan calmly stated her point of view. She said that Fred had had a passion for food all of his life. He looked forward to mealtimes and as his health deteriorated this became one of his only pleasures. Joan said that she didn't expect any of us to understand but she knew her husband and what he would want. She told us that she couldn't give her husband much any more but she could take a stand and make sure that at least he had nice food to eat. She added almost cynically, "If he dies choking, at least it will be something worth choking on - not just a pile of mush." The staff told Joan in no uncertain terms that they did not want to be responsible for Fred choking whilst one of them was feeding him. Joan said that she would take that responsibility as his next of kin and was willing to put it in writing.

The outcome was that when Joan was there, he was given solid food but when she wasn't the staff fed Fred liquidised food. Somehow I pacified myself with the thought that the staff were only doing it for Fred's own good, yet I knew in my heart that what we were doing was wrong.'

This is an example of an ethical dilemma related to risk management that happens every day in practice but in this case it was 'covered up' or 'managed'. The key issue for us in this story is the nature of true partnerships - if we are to work together with clients and their families an open and honest approach has to be used so that a solution based on mutual trust is found. Even if an intervention is perceived by staff as being in the best interest of the patient, there is a danger of trust being shattered if the foundation for that trust is built on pretence.

Using guidelines and reports to inform practice

The NMC Code: *Standards of conduct, performance and ethics* (2008) recognises the importance of partnerships in care based on informed choice and the patient's right to decide whether or not to undergo any health-care intervention. It states that 'Nurses must listen and respond to the concerns and preferences of people in their care' (NMC 2008:3). Various government policies have also promoted patient choice and control over services (Department of Heath, 2001, 2005, 2007) with autonomy and advocacy seen as key issues. However, these aspects need to be carefully considered so that mutually acceptable solutions to problems are arrived at. This may involve mediation with carers. UKCC (1998)

Guidelines for Mental Health and Learning Disabilities Nursing also recognised the difficulties inherent within the client–professional power balance.

> *'You must not practise in a way which assumes that only you know what is best for a client. This may create dependency, hinders teamwork and can interfere with the client's right to choose. Some clients may be highly suggestible and thus more likely to agree to suggestions or choices from those in positions of authority. Advocacy is about promoting clients' rights to choose and empowering them to decide for themselves.'*
> *(UKCC, 1998:14)*

Skidmore (2005:25) suggests that there is a place for the expert professional in giving advice but not to act as a 'life director'. 'The expert should use their expertise to facilitate another's journey; be it through health, education or the workplace. To do otherwise removes control from the individual and makes them forever dependent upon the "expert".'

People with learning disabilities may become particularly powerless because of the way they are perceived and this may have a disastrous effect on any care or treatment they receive. The *Treat Me Right!* report from Mencap in 2004 highlighted the unequal health care that they often receive from health-care professionals and this was reiterated by the Disability Rights Commission in 2006, which published the results of a formal investigation into physical health inequalities experienced by people with learning disabilities and mental health problems. A Mencap report that followed on from this, entitled *Death by Indifference* and published in 2007, claimed 'institutional discrimination' within the NHS and included case studies outlining the traumatic experiences of six people who died whilst in hospital care. A common complaint of their families was that they felt consistently ignored when they expressed their concerns. The report called for improved staff training to reduce the risk of diagnostic overshadowing which is explained as the belief that 'a presenting problem is a feature of someone's learning disability and that not much can be done about it' (Mencap, 2007: 20). As we have seen, nurses have an important role to play in listening to families and getting their help in recognising important, and perhaps to us uncommon, indications of problems. We need to be aware that family members or other carers can play a key role in interpreting distress cues and other signs and behaviour that might be missed by professional staff.

The need for anti-discriminatory practice

Although there is a particular problem for people with learning disabilities, there is also a danger in letting our assumptions misinterpret important cues with other client groups. Some people have great insights into the way stock answers are sometimes used to 'reassure' patients and dismiss their concerns. Jasmin, a student nurse, told us how much she learned from Gordon, a 75-year-old man who asked a doctor undertaking his ward round to look at his very painful knee.

'Don't worry about it,' the doctor said sympathetically; 'it's just old age.'

'Well,' said Gordon, 'the other knee's the same age but that isn't giving me any problem!'

We need to be very careful that we listen to what people are saying and that we do not discount it by interpreting it as entirely due to some pre-existing condition such as age or disability. The NMC (2009) published guidance for care of older people and emphasised the nurse's responsibility to ensure that the care received by older people is of a consistently high standard, whether it is provided by oneself, a colleague or someone to whom you have delegated care. It states that nurses should be continually monitoring and challenging if poor care is provided by colleagues and championing the quality of each older person's care experience. The report stresses the importance of giving feedback to colleagues on their competence in caring, especially in relation to their behaviour and attitude. Negative stereotypical views about older people are likely to result in undignified, neglectful or abusive care. The report, based on experiences of older people gives an example of this: 'A nurse said "You're not getting back into bed until you eat this," but I couldn't eat it so I had to sit there. My legs were killing me' (2009:13).

People with mental health problems sometimes face prejudice when accessing health services. Assumptions made about them may interfere with diagnosis but may more commonly be associated with reactions of indifference or frustration. Hilary, a student nurse, wrote of her concern about the way Jason was treated in an A+E department. Consider and reflect on this account.

Case Study 3.12

'The paramedics brought in Jason who claimed he had taken 45 co-codamol tablets with alcohol. They handed him over to my mentor, who looked at Jason sitting in the corridor and said to me, "Do that man's observations, please, and take him to the assessment room" (this is where the psychological assessments are carried out). I was very shocked and confused by his attitude towards Jason. My mentor did not communicate with Jason at all, which was out of character for him. I walked over to Jason and explained I was going to take his temperature and blood pressure. As I was applying the cuff he began to cry. I did not know what to say to him and was worried in case I said the wrong thing and upset him further so I smiled sympathetically and touched him on the arm but I did not know whether that was the right thing to do or not. After I'd finished the observations I escorted him to the assessment room. I asked Jason if he was all right and if he wanted anything and then went back to inform my mentor about the observations I had taken. My mentor explained that Jason was a "regular attender" at the A+E, often attending after taking an overdose. This seemed to anger my mentor. I could not understand why he felt this way as there must be a reason why Jason kept trying to commit suicide. I was shocked that, although he was treated for his overdose, no member of staff showed they cared about Jason or talked to him as a person. They seemed to be wanting to get him out of the A+E as quickly as possible.'

Time to think back

+ How would you describe the attitudes of the staff in the accident and emergency department?
+ How did these attitudes influence their behaviour towards Jason?
+ What effect did the experience have on Hilary?
+ Do you know of any theoretical perspectives, guidelines or reports that might have informed practice?

Compare your findings with ours

Jason's presence in A+E seems to have evoked strong feelings of anger and perhaps frustration. He was the subject of stereotyping by Hilary's mentor (a generalisation that he belonged to a group of 'regular attenders', seen as having certain characteristics). This stereotyping may have led to the belief that people who self-harmed 'wasted staff time' and were themselves to blame for their actions (negative prejudice). This may have resulted in discrimination, in that there may have been inappropriate or inadequate care for Jason. You may have thought that in this case the mentor demonstrated this by avoiding Jason's care and leaving it to Hilary, who was inexperienced and finding it very difficult to know how best to communicate with him. She needed guidance and reassurance from a mentor who needed to review his own approach, not only to Jason but also to Hilary, perhaps through gaining more guidance and support for himself. You may have in your reflections, psychological or sociological literature or nursing resources that have helped you to understand these key concepts in more depth.

You may have included guidelines from the National Institute for Clinical Excellence (NICE), which were developed in 2004 in response to the 'unacceptable' and sometimes punitive treatment of the large number of people who deliberately injure themselves. These guidelines emphasised the need for health-care professionals to show compassion and understanding, take account of the likely distress associated with self-harm and ensure that people who self-harm are adequately assessed. They should be asked to explain their feelings and understandings in their own words, in a private and safe environment. The guidelines go on to say that 'In caring for people who repeatedly self-harm, health care professionals should be aware that the individual's reasons for self-harming may be different on each occasion and therefore each episode needs to be treated in its own right' (NICE, 2004:8). In Jason's case the mentor did not seem willing to do this. However, there is also recognition of the stress and demands of caring for people who self-harm. The report acknowledges that providing treatment and care for them is emotionally demanding and it suggests that all staff involved in this kind of work should have regular supervision so that they can explore its emotional impact on them. Hilary was surprised because the reaction to Jason by her mentor seemed out of character, so it seems likely that he needs support so that he has a chance to talk through his negativity and gain more understanding and guidance.

We have talked about the importance of empathy, but as we struggle with difficult situations, the need to be caring can make heavy demands on us. According to Salvage (2006:22), this is not just being polite or superficially pleasant. She writes: 'The genuine empathy that generates compassionate action is creative and challenging, not the sugary sort of niceness so often linked with the traditional image of nursing.' This may be particularly challenging when people such as Jason present us with difficult problems for which we can see little solution. However, if we are to be truly caring, we need to find ways in which to contain our frustrations and misgivings and learn to work with them so that we can ease, rather than increase, their problems.

To do this we must be able to identify and learn to overcome the prejudices that are part of all of us. At times these may be because of lack of knowledge or familiarity concerning people from a particular culture, for example black or ethnic minority groups. We may also make false assumptions and develop misunderstandings about people with particular conditions or histories, or those who belong to different religions, groups or backgrounds from us. These prejudices can lead to uncaring attitudes and behaviours and are against the NMC

Code (2008), which you should have included in your reflections since this is the code out-lining standards for conduct, performance and ethics, under which we must all practise. For example, the code instructs us to make the care of people our first concern by treating them as individuals and respecting their dignity.

Working together

People with long-term conditions are also in particular need of good working relationships with health-care professionals. The code of conduct highlights the importance of collaborating with those in our care. Recognition of the knowledge and skills of people with long-term condi-tions has been acknowledged by the Department of Health, (2001) in its document entitled *The Expert Patient: A new approach to chronic disease management for the twenty-first century.* This report advocated a shift towards more equal partnerships between service users and pro-fessionals in working together and gaining more understanding about how people can best manage chronic conditions.

Creating a 'patient-led' NHS is a high priority, and within acute and community care settings the need for greater responsiveness to users' needs and flexibility in the way in which care is provided is gaining greater momentum(e.g. Department of Health, 2009). Many patients have extensive experience of a variety of hospitals and wards, making them 'experts' in evaluating what caring really means. If no one listens to patients with experi-ence or their relatives or if they are too frightened to say what they really think of the care they receive, we will be unable to draw directly on this expertise. Toni, who has lived for years with chronic asthma, reflected on one of her admissions to a particular hospital in this way:

> 'I was frightened to say too much because of possible repercussions. ... I will never go back to that hospital. I believe they could have killed me – they didn't listen to what my husband said had helped before. I did not complain directly. But when the hospital posted me a questionnaire I completed it because I could remain anonymous.'

A culture of open dialogue must be created so any misconceptions can be clarified, fears reduced, assumptions challenged and immediate action taken when required. Stories or incidents from practice, particularly if they are apparently critical of care, are sometimes criticised for being individual perspectives and therefore may be considered not to be truly representative. However, we are suggesting that by using incidents such as those included above, much may be learned about how actions are perceived. Realistically, people do make mistakes, are sometimes hard to communicate with or have particular behaviours or characteristics that we dislike or with which we disagree. However, we must enter into a dialogue with them so that we understand their preoccupations and concerns and also, most importantly, try to help them to understand us. 'The patient experience is constructed and shaped through dialogue; it is only in the sharing of the experience that it is (trans)formed into knowledge' (Rolfe, 2005:xiii). Reflecting on dis-tressing incidents told to us by patients and also staff will help us not only to take action if necessary but also to gain understanding and free us from unthinking and discrimina-tory practices.

Summary

In this chapter we have considered the need for putting more compassion into care. We have looked at both caring and uncaring moments in practice. The stories we have chosen of uncaring or negative attitudes may have not led to official complaints or investigations into professional misconduct but have been the kinds of events that can occur almost every day in practice and are mainly the result of unthinking or uninformed care rather than deliberate cruelty. Nevertheless, in some cases they cause extreme distress and may have long-term effects on service users and their families. We have seen that to overcome such difficulties we need to focus on:

+ Developing a heightened awareness by listening to and 'hearing' patients' lived experiences.
+ Simple acts of kindness that may be easily overlooked, hidden and undervalued.
+ Showing compassion, developing and using skills of reassurance and empathy.
+ Being proactive about care needs.
+ Being aware of our own assumptions and promoting and engaging in anti-discriminatory practice.
+ Working in partnership, including acknowledging the contribution of the patient with experience.
+ Raising any concerns related to poor-quality care.

Looking forward

The impact of caring in terms of the nurse's emotional involvement cannot be underestimated, particularly given the unpredictable and sometimes distressing nature of nursing care. As we have seen in this chapter, there are situations that are challenging and require the expenditure of considerable emotional energy, sometimes known as 'labour'. These aspects and professional boundaries which need to be taken into account will be explored within the next chapter.

Activity

+ Reflect on your care and consider whether you have made assumptions about the people you have cared for.
+ Have you had to revise your views in the light of experience?
+ What has that taught you about your future practice?
+ Use the indicators below to see how they can help you to engage in anti-discriminatory, caring practice.

Caring indicators

1. Attending to fundamental care needs such as hygiene, nutrition, pain relief, promoting dignity and comfort

2. Demonstrating high level/mastery of technical skills, but using these while delivering care in a holistic and empathic manner

3. Creating a culture of trust, honesty and open dialogue with patients and carers so that they feel able to voice their feelings, preferences and experiences

4. Communicating sensitively and effectively, listening to and exchanging information and knowledge with patients and carers, overcoming any barriers so they can make their feelings and needs known

5. Being proactive, by asking patients what they need and responding to cues; not waiting to be asked or making assumptions

6. Using and developing skills of empathy, taking into account professional boundaries

7. Engaging in simple acts of kindness, showing regard and respect for others, promoting positive self-esteem

8. Providing effective, therapeutic reassurance

9. Respecting others by engaging in anti-discriminatory practice, irrespective of their age, gender, cultural origins, class, status or condition from which they suffer

10. Monitoring the quality of care provided by yourself or those to whom you have delegated care and reporting any concerns you might have

References

Age Concern (2006) Hungry to be Heard: The scandal of malnourished older people in hospital. London: Age Concern.

Bartlett, A (2011) *Making intentional rounding happen.* Paper presented at 'Transforming patient experience conference'. Available at: **www.kingsfund.org.uk.** (last accessed 13/02/2112).

Buber, M (1958) *I and Thou.* New York: Scribner.

Burnell, L (2009) Compassionate care; a concept analysis. *Home Health Care Management and Practice, 21,5,319-324.*

Care Quality Commission (2011) *State of Care Report 2010-2011* Available at: **www.cqc.org.uk.** (last accessed 13/02/2011).

Chambers, C and Ryder, E (2009) *Compassion and Caring in Nursing. Oxon:* Radcliffe Publishing Ltd.

Cornwell, J and Goodrich, J (2008) Seeing the person in the patient. Point of care review paper. London: King's Fund.

Davies, D (2007) Reflection on practice: an intubated patient suffering panic attacks. *Nursing in Critical Care* **12**, 198-201.

Davison, N, Williams, K (2009) Compassion in nursing 1: defining, identifying and measuring this essential quality. *Nursing Times*; 105: 36, 16-18.

Department of Health (2001) The Expert Patient: *A new approach to chronic disease management for the twenty-first century*. London: Stationery Office.

Department of Health (2006) *A new ambition for old age: Next Steps in Implementing the National Service Frameworks for Older People*. London: Stationery Office.

Department of Health (2007) *Our NHS, Our Future*. Interim Report. London: Stationery Office.

Department of Health (2008) *Confidence in caring: a framework for best practice*. Available at: **www. dh.gov.uk.** (last accessed 22 /01/ 2012).

Department of Health (2009) *Understanding what matters: a guide to using patient feedback to transform care*. Available at: **www.dh.gov.uk.** (last accessed 16/02/ 2012).

Department of Health (2012) *The NHS Constitution for England*. Available at: **www.dh.gov.uk/ publications**. (last accessed 13/02/2012).

Dignity in Care Campaign. Available at: **www.dignityincare.org.uk** (last accessed 13/02/2012).

Disability Rights Commission (2006) *Equal Treatment: Closing the gap. A formal investigation into the physical health inequalities experienced by people with learning disabilities and/or mental health problems*. London Disability Rights Commission.

Egan, G (2001) (7th edition) *The Skilled Helper* Bevery, MA: Wadsworth Publishing Co.Inc.

Francis, R (2010) Independent Inquiry into care provided by Mid-Staffordshire NHS Foundation Trust January 2005–March 2009. London: Stationery Office.

Goffman, E (1969) *The Presentation of Self in Everyday Life*. Harmondsworth: Penguin.

Great Britain, Parliamentary and Health Service Ombudsman (2011) *Care and compassion? Report of the Health service Ombudsman on 10 investigations into NHS care of older people*. London: Stationery Office.

McCabe, C (2004) Nurse–patient communication: an exploration of patients' experiences *Journal of Clinical Nursing* **13**, 41–49.

Mencap (2004) *Treat Me Right!* London: Mencap.

Mencap (2007) *Death by Indifference Report*. London: Mencap.

MIND (2012) *Listening to experience. Independent inquiry into acute and crisis mental health care*. Available at: **www.mind.org.uk.** (last accessed 09/02/2012).

National Institute for Clinical Excellence (2004) *The short-term physical and psychological management and secondary prevention of self-harm in primary and secondary care. Clinical Guidelines* **16**. London: NICE. Available at: **www.nice.org.uk.** (last accessed 13/04/2012).

National Pensioners Convention (2112) *Dignity Code*. Available at: **www.npcuk.org.** (last accessed 24/02/2112).

Noddings, N (2003) *'Caring' a feminine approach to ethics and moral education*. Berkeley CA: University of California Press.

NMC (Nursing and Midwifery Council) (2008) *The Code: Standards of conduct, performance and ethics for nurses and midwives*. London: Nursing and Midwifery Council.

NMC (2009) *Guidance for the care of older people*. Available at: **www.nmc.org.uk** (last accessed 13/04/2012).

NMC (2010) *Raising and escalating concerns: Guidance for nurses and midwives*. London: Nursing and Midwifery Council.

Nussbaum M (2001) *Upheavals of thought*. Cambridge: Cambridge University Press.

Parker, V (1999) On confronting life and death. In Madjar, I and Walton, J (eds) *Nursing and the Experience of Illness Phenomenology in Practice*. London: Routledge.

Patients Association (2011) *Care Campaign*. Available at: **www.Patients-association.com** (last accessed 13/04/2012).

Price, B (2004) Demonstrating respect for patient dignity. *Nursing Standard* **19**, 45-51.

Rogers, C R (1991) *Client-centred Therapy*. London: Constable.

Rolfe, G (2005) Foreword. In Warne, T and McAndrew, S (eds) *Using Patient Experience in Nurse Education*. Basingstoke: Palgrave Macmillan.

Salvage, J (2006) It's the action that counts. *Nursing Standard* **20**, 20-23.

Schantz, M (2007) Compassion: a concept analysis. *Nursing Forum;* **42**: 2, 48-55.

Skidmore, D (2005) The person as a life expert: this is not a love song. In Warne, T and McAndrew, S (eds) *Using Patient Experience in Nurse Education*. Basingstoke: Palgrave Macmillan.

Smith, Stevie (1981) Not waving but drowning. In Smith, S *Collected Poems*. New York: New Directions Publishing Corporation.

Teasdale, K (1995) Theoretical and practical considerations on the use of reassurance in the management of anxious patients. *Journal of Advanced Nursing* **22**, 79-86.

UKCC (UK Central Council for Nursing, Midwifery and Health Visiting) (1998) *Guidelines for Mental Health and Learning Disabilities Nursing*. London: UK Central Council for Nursing, Midwifery and Health Visiting.

Van der Cingel, M (2011) Compassion in care: A qualitative study of older people with a chronic disease and nurses *Nursing Ethics* **18**(5) 672-685.

Warne, T and McAndrew, S (eds) (2005) *Using Patient Experience in Nurse Education*. Basingstoke: Palgrave Macmillan.

West, L (2006) Student experiences in the real world of nursing. Starting out. *Nursing Standard* **20**, 29.

Wilkin, K and Slevin, E (2004) The meaning of caring to nurses: an investigation into the nature of caring work in an intensive care unit. *Journal of Clinical Nursing* **13**, 50-59 51.

Williams, A and Irurita, V (2006) Emotional comfort: The patient's perspective of a therapeutic context. *International Journal of Nursing Studies* **43**, 405-415.

Wynne-Jones, M (2006) The patient who won't be reassured. *Pulse* **37**, 72.

Younger, R (2008) *Compassion in health care*. NHS Confederation Futures debates. Available at: **www.nhsconfed.org/Publications/Pages/Compassion-in-healthcare.aspx** (last accessed 17/03/2012).

Chapter 4

Bonds, boundaries and balance in the emotional world of nursing

LEARNING OBJECTIVES

By the end of this chapter you should have an understanding of:

1. How emotions may affect care in practice including judgements and behaviour

2. Emotional labour as an essential part of caring

3. How identification with particular patients can affect our emotional balance

4. The boundaries of the professional relationship

5. The importance of using opportunities for reflective learning

Introduction

In this chapter we will further explore how emotions affect our practice. Compassionate care involves assisting in ways that are beneficial to service users and their families. However, it is important to see how to maintain a balance so that we neither distance ourselves (nor perhaps be perceived as lacking compassion) or become so overwhelmed that we cannot help effectively. Nurses are often witness to traumatic, life-changing events and are also undertaking complex (and often undervalued) caring needs of vulnerable people with long-term disabilities. They need to respond quickly to acute and unpredictable situations and also to cope with everyday demands on them as they try to be physically and psychologically available to others. So nursing is far from an easy job.

Incidents and scenarios we have collected from our student nurse workshops indicate that, from the very beginning, it is important for students to explore the parameters, rules or boundaries of their work. The students' stories clearly show that they can be very uneasy about what it might mean to really care, how much emotional involvement there ought to be with clients and their families and how different types of emotional involvement (or otherwise) can affect themselves and their clients. Our students raised numerous questions about their concerns; for example: Should I attend the funerals of people I particularly care for? Where does my responsibility end? How should I feel about this? Am I a bad person if I don't get upset at something that others find harrowing? What am I to do with these guilty feelings? When I feel overwhelmed by events, should I try to shut off from emotional involvement? Why do I feel so guilty if I cannot give the amount of care I would like? These are just a few of the questions that caused anxiety for a large number of our student nurses. If you are a qualified nurse you may recognise these responses and may still feel uneasy about similar issues.

In this chapter we will explore some of these questions and again use stories to help us see the kinds of experiences that can have an emotional impact on nurses.

Caring for people – emotional work

Nursing is not just a series of tasks that have to be undertaken in a prescribed time frame, although it may seem like this at times. Read Andy's story to see how a qualified mental health nurse reminded himself of the most important focus of his work.

Case Study 4.1

'As a community psychiatric nurse (CPN) for the older person I had a lot of new referrals to visit. It was a Monday morning and there had been a heavy snowfall the night before. I was very keen to start seeing these new clients, but had to see Terry, a 65-year-old. I noticed the path had been cleared. Thinking it was Terry who had done this, I called out "Who's been busy this morning then?" It was his brother. Terry had died that morning, clearing the path, due to a heart attack. I stayed and spoke to his family.

On leaving the village I saw a funeral car arriving at the home of a woman I had visited recently and who had then been admitted to the psychiatric hospital. She had died there but I had not been informed. I called to see the family.

Driving back, I reflected that earlier that morning I had felt "bogged down" with the physical aspects of my work and the problems. The events of the morning brought it back to me that primarily I deal with, and get to know, people. I was not so hassled that week, reminding myself of this.'

Reflecting back on two unexpected deaths caused Andy to pause and review what his work was really about. His relationship with both patients' families prompted him to demonstrate a caring attitude and acknowledge the importance of their loss. Andy was an experienced nurse and was able to find his own particular way of effectively coping with any sadness he might have felt. He seems not to have become hardened to the death of his clients and saw his care of relatives as an important part of that care. Andy gave us this incident at a reflective workshop for qualified nurses, when he chose to look back at the importance of his feelings. Andy, like many nurses however experienced they are, finds 'debriefing' (or talking over the situation with supportive others) beneficial after such an event. Parkinson (1997) argues that this helps to 'normalise' emotions, making individuals aware that their feelings are normal for what they have experienced. This is important since Smith (1992:96) suggests that death and dying can call for 'the ultimate emotional labour'.

Linking theory to practice

You might have noticed that Andy said that he had been 'bogged down' with the physical aspects of his work. However, he realised the importance of the emotional side of his work in caring for people. In Chapter 1 we discussed the view that the demands of emotional work can be as hard as physical and technical labour. Sociologists such as Strauss et al. (1982) and James (1992) have emphasised the importance of taking this into account since it has implications for both carer and the person being cared for. They suggest that changes in modern medicine have led to a shift in emphasis from holistic regard for the individual to a biomedical model with a focus on the diagnosis and treatment of physiological malfunctioning of particular organs or systems. However, the success of modern health care in terms of the use of technology and a range of medical interventions and drugs has meant an increase in the complexity of the care provided and in the skills required to do it. Such care has overshadowed and devalued emotional care although there is evidence of its increasing importance. Phillips (1996) sees the value of this in terms of providing reassurance and support, not just to ensure compliance but also in helping the overall psychological and physical well-being of the patient. The effect of emotional labour on health-care professionals was also recognised by James (1992) who saw it as difficult, personal, often upsetting and requiring a great deal of thought, skill and time.

Acknowledgement of the need to provide emotional support as part of holistic-centred care has been recognised in strategies employed by nurses such as individualised care plans, models of nursing and the named or primary nurse. All of these strategies depend on careful implementation and evaluation. In holistic care, psychological, social, spiritual as well as physiological needs are taken into account. However, because of the low status of emotional work there may be little support for what may sometimes be a complex task, taking time and energy. For example, in a busy ward, particularly when caring for vulnerable patients, it is often quicker and easier for the nurse to take over the care instead of encouraging independence. This can lead to feelings of disempowerment and loss of identity so that service users become passive and dependent – indications of poor-quality care. Chambers and Ryder (2009:171) emphasise the dangers of this, asserting 'We need to challenge passive, discouraging and disempowering behaviour in others at all times and take action so that does not become common practice, or embedded into the culture of the organisation or practice area.' Research by Mackintosh (2006) on the professional socialisation of nurses confirms that the culture of an organisation is in danger of doing this by encouraging nurses to maintain emotional distance and prioritise practical tasks. An alternative culture of compassionate caring is therefore essential and depends on effective leadership and management so that individualised care is not just rhetoric but reality.

Emotional care involves gaining knowledge of service users' concerns, preferences and perspectives if interventions are to be effective, so that trust is created and partnerships can be fostered. In relation to this, Dizon (2007), speaking in a World Health Organization conference on the promotion of people-centred care, highlighted the importance of nurses throughout the world:

> 'The nurse's role as the "front-liner" in patient care continues to be of primary importance. Nurses spend the most time with the patient for the duration of his or her stay in hospital. The attention they provide, or the lack of it, constitutes the patient's lasting impression about his or her hospital experience. Thus, the patient's perception of the expertise, skill and empathy of the nurse is valuable in the care cycle. Nurses have always been the principal advocates for safe and compassionate care.'

However, as indicated in Chapter 3, there is much evidence to suggest that although safe and compassionate care has been the cornerstone of nursing in the UK, at present the profession is going through a time of change and increasing demands and challenges have led to some loss of public confidence in the degree to which compassion is still there in nursing. There are therefore important questions to ask, including how, in spite of the challenges inherent in a complex and at times overstretched health-care system, nurses can learn about and maintain compassion in their care and how stress-related responses that have a derogatory effect on the quality of care such as 'compassion fatigue' can be avoided.

There is a strong argument that nurses need more time to show they 'care about' as well as 'care for' patients but also an acknowledgment that students and nurses at all levels need to be able to talk about their experiences, particularly those they find upsetting. In her study of student nurses' experiences, Smith (1992:110) commented that there was:

> 'an expectation that the more senior a student was the more likely she would be expected to cope with upsetting situations. It seemed that because students' feelings were rarely acknowledged in the open arena of the ward they were likely to develop distancing strategies that kept them from personal involvement. They recognised that, as they progressed through their careers, they might become hard. But they also recognised that if they hardened and distanced too much they would be unable to nurse with feeling.'

Reflection can help us to acknowledge and work with our feelings about events.

To think about

Think of an incident from practice that has had an emotional impact on you and analyse it. We have chosen a framework developed by Smith and Russell (1991), which was slightly amended by Schutz, Angove and Sharp (2004:58) to help you do this:

+ Write a description of the incident.
+ Outline why you chose the event and how and why it is significant for you.
+ Identify any key issues (perhaps questions that emerge) and why they are important.
+ Reflect on:
    - How you were involved, why and what you felt.
    - Why you behaved the way you did and how you made your decisions.
    - The part that others played and why you think they behaved as they did.
    - What else was happening in the context at the time.
    - The relevant theoretical background.
    - What action might be indicated either now or in the future.
    - How you evaluate what happened in terms of what you have learned in a specific and in a general sense.

As a student you might like to keep this information within a reflective learning diary or to inform your ongoing assessment record. If you are a mentor you might assist your student with this or use it to provide a focus for discussion about emotional boundaries within compassionate care.

The analysis may have uncovered uncomfortable or confusing feelings. Using the framework may have helped you to clarify your thinking, emotions and perhaps your behaviour. It is not an easy task to be self-aware but you will find it can help to bring out the positive as well as the negative ways in which you and others respond to situations. The framework also points out that you should consider the effect of your reflections on your actions in the future. This questioning approach is essential in order for you to continue to develop personally and professionally. We all need to think critically about our practice in order to learn and develop from it. It is a never-ending quest throughout our professional lives and the emotional as well as the technical skills acquired as a student will shape the nurse of the future.

Managing emotions

There is a need, if we want to be truly caring and effective, to find some sort of balance between being neither 'overemotional' nor blasé. The following stories give you an idea of some of the difficulties associated with managing feelings about an aspect that we may find particularly problematic – caring for the dying. They also demonstrate that an opportunity to discuss incidents and feelings with others is beneficial and supportive. Staff nurses at a mentor workshop noted that every experience of caring for dying patients and their relatives was unique and, even if expected, could result in vividly retained memories.

Case Study 4.2

'A lady died in the ward. My student had never seen a dead body before so I realised it was going to be hard . . . During the coffee break I took the opportunity to talk things over with her. There were a few of us who were talking about our experiences and we said, "Oh God, do you remember the first time we saw anybody die or have an arrest?" "Yes, I'll never forget the first woman I saw dead. Not that it was a horrible experience. It wasn't; just one that's always going to stay with me."

I think a student is often facing new experiences and we had a particularly horrible death not so long ago. That is not a very nice way of putting it, but it was a stressful death for the few students that were around . . . A student had been there when the wife ran out of the room screaming as he arrested. So she basically got it "full on". I thought that it was really important for someone to go through that with her because the wife was still hysterical over an hour later. This guy was young!'

The above incidents show that the mentors were sensitive to the needs and feelings of students. They empathised with the students and used their own past experiences to help them. Being able to talk over events meant the staff were also able to consider their own feelings and reactions to the dying patients and their families. This is an example of the importance of passing on 'tacit' knowledge that is often hidden, or embedded, within nursing and that you may not find in your textbooks. In this case the mentors shared their knowledge and experiences of how to deal with such difficult situations in practice. They recognised the importance of helping students with the 'emotional labour' associated with death and this is important as it is likely to strike a chord within us, for example, regarding our own mortality and the transient nature of all human beings.

Connecting with a dying patient

Read the traumatic incident below, written by a third-year student nurse, and consider why it was particularly emotional for her.

Case Study 4.3

'On a night shift we received a trauma call at approximately one in the morning. We were informed that we were to receive a young male with multiple stab wounds. In response we put out a trauma call. This requires a member from each discipline to attend A+E should their expertise be required, for instance anaesthetics, surgery, orthopaedics and the night sister. We prepared ourselves for the arrival of the patient, we wore apron and gloves, linked up the ambu bag to the oxygen, ran some fluid through ready and set up the trauma sheet and then we stood waiting.

On arrival of the young man, the paramedics instructed us that the most severe wounds were on his back but we soon realised that his puncture wounds were everywhere. He had a large slit from his mouth up his cheek, which was horrible. He also had puncture wounds to his arms and hands, probably from where he had lifted his hands to try to protect himself.

We immediately rolled him onto his side and took down the paramedics' dressing to assess the severity of the wounds to his back. There were three severe stab wounds to his back. The sister dressed them with a pressure dressing. Fluids were commenced and regular blood pressure results were monitored. He was conscious with a Glasgow Coma Score (GCS) of 15/15. He constantly asked for our names. With each new set of hands he felt touch him he asked who it was and what their name was. He was so grateful and kept saying "Thank you, if the paramedics hadn't got there when they did I would be dead now, wouldn't I?"

He had an oxygen mask on but the doctors decided that he required chest drains. It was all happening so fast that I'm not sure why he needed them, whether it was because he wasn't saturating enough, or his chest wasn't rising properly or whether it was due to the area in his back that the stab wounds were; I am honestly unsure. They decided to put bilateral chest drains in and whilst the left-sided chest drain went in relatively easily, the doctor carrying out the right-sided chest drain initially had some difficulty getting it in. They asked me to hold his hands while they put the chest drains in. This was probably partly for some reassurance, but also to literally hold his hands down to prevent him from pushing his hands up to stop the painful stimulus of inserting the drains. Even in pain he was much stronger than I was. I held his hand and he asked me my name, and said it was nice to meet me. I replied that it was nice to meet him too. He squeezed my hand and I squeezed his hand back. As I did so my finger seemed to disappear, it had sunk into one of the wounds in his hands. They were bleeding badly. Sister seemed to notice the blood loss at the same time as I did and I suggested we dress his hand. She agreed and held his hand up off the bed to enable me to dress it. He was transferred to theatre.

I had to go and attend to the rest of A+E, which was extremely busy . . . The department was packed and we had to continue attending to other patients but we all kept making comments about how we wondered how he was and informing each other of any news. It was a waiting game. Just before 7 a.m. the theatre staff came to retrieve his family. He was dying and they took them to be with him for his last few minutes. They escorted them to the recovery room. It was so horrible! I had a numb feeling afterwards . . . '

Case Study 4.4

Compare your considerations with part of the student's explanation of her feelings below. Note the way she uses theory to help her to do this.

'. . . It would be fair to say that I myself had become blasé in dealing with trauma situations as they had never affected me personally before. Rather interestingly, Gibson and Iwaniec (2003) point out that the word 'trauma' comes from the Greek and means 'to pierce or puncture armour'. They state that it is important to consider this when preparing helpers to face incidents that have the potential for piercing their usual coping strategies. It is clear that my own coping strategies appear to have suffered a similar assault with regard to this incident.

The reason for my feeling so emotionally involved has still probably not been clarified. It was due to a number of reasons. The patient was about the same age as me . . . More important, though, was the fact that he knew my name and I had held his hand through a dreadfully painful and frightening ordeal. It was through these two simple forms of communication, in this intense situation, that I felt as though we had made some kind of connection. Although it sounds extremely overdramatic, in the immediate aftermath of that incident I recognised that there had been an almost spiritual connection. The need for him to know people's names suggests a need to know the people around him, to give him some security and comfort in his time of need.

Ronaldson (2000) describes moments such as these as times of spiritual searching and intensity which may occur in the hustle and bustle of everyday care. She states that nurses are involved in patients' spirituality every time we practise and our own spirituality is affected. Similarly, Eastbrooks and Morse (1992) state that the final phase of connection with a patient is touching, which they suggest is more than just the skin-to-skin contact. One informant actually described the completion of touching as "bumping souls". This is something similar to what I personally felt in the aftermath of the trauma . . .'

This moving reflective account helps us to understand the student's intense feelings in a traumatic situation and shows how she contributed with compassion to the care the young man received. She needed to explore the intensity of her emotions both verbally with her tutor and then further in a written form. She was able to make more sense of her experience by using a variety of perspectives, so this is an excellent example of how vital reflection can be. Her emotional and academic labour became an important resource in helping her to develop both personally and professionally.

The part identification may play in our emotional reactions

In an earlier chapter we described the sense of connection or identification we can have with particular patients and their families when we feel as if 'a button is pressed within us' and we feel especially linked to them. This can enable us to connect with them very quickly but can also uncover deep emotions within us. Some situations may be more significant and even problematic for us because they remind us of someone we love, perhaps someone who has died, and so we associate our feelings of loss with them. It may also make us more aware of our own mortality, for example, if they are of a similar age to us. The triggers for these emotions may be very unexpected, as you will discover in the next incident, written by Janice.

Case Study 4.5

'. . . the paramedics informed us that they were approaching the hospital with a patient who had undergone a cardiac arrest. Immediately my heart started to race as I had no previous experience of the situation and did not know what to expect. Initially I was excited and could not wait to witness such a new experience. The staff nurse and I made our way to the designated area and prepared for the arrival of the patient. At that time my main concern was that I would be asked to participate in the process and, to be honest, I did not give much thought to the fact that this was a person with a life and a family. When the patient arrived the staff nurse proceeded with basic life support and the doctor administered a drug. After approximately 10 minutes of witnessing this, I thought about what I was seeing and silently congratulated myself on handling the situation so well. Suddenly I stopped looking at the patient and looked at 'John'. He had the exact same pair of slippers on as my granddad wears. Well, that was it! I felt very sad and saw him as a person in his own right rather than just a patient who was receiving medical attention – I could easily have burst into tears right then and actively controlled the urge to get upset.'

Time to think back

+ How did Janice's emotions and thoughts change over the short period described?
+ What was the trigger that changed her feelings about John?
+ What was the benefit of the 'trigger' and what were the consequences of its impact on her?
+ What could have helped her cope with the situation?

It must have been very difficult for Janice to control her feelings, but given that she was involved in caring for a patient in a life-threatening situation as part of the team, she showed selflessness in controlling her feelings although we know that she found it helpful to talk about these intense feelings at a later time. All nurses may experience these unexpected triggers although they may be hidden from our immediate awareness. We will go on to discuss these issues further.

Suzie, a newly qualified nurse, had a similar experience to Janice. Consider the following incident and jot down anything you think might have had an effect on her emotional state (consciously or unconsciously).

Case Study 4.6

'I was working on the accident and emergency department. I came on duty at 4 p.m. on Easter Sunday. I had spent the afternoon with my four-year-old niece, opening Easter eggs and generally enjoying a great afternoon.

On arrival in the department I was confronted with the grieving parents of a three-year-old girl, who had died by choking on a plastic toy from inside one of her eggs. I was told by the senior nurse to stay with the parents in the interview room and that they would want to see their child again. I felt very nervous because I had secretly avoided grieving relatives in the past and I now felt I did not have the special skills to deal with distressed relatives.

> The parents were recently separated. The father of the child was aggressive and rather hysterical. Although I felt completely out of my depth and just did not know what to say, I stayed with them. The final stressor came when I accompanied the parents to see their daughter. She was wearing white socks with red hearts on them and they were the same as the ones my niece was wearing when I had left her an hour before.

Compare your considerations with ours

Suzie went from a happy scenario at home into a sad and distressing one at work. The closeness and immediacy of two contrasting environments that were connected by similarities (e.g. similar children, Easter eggs, and same patterned socks) made a particular impact. She was faced with the need to cope with grieving relatives – the father was described as 'aggressive' and 'hysterical'. She highlights the fact that she had avoided grieving relatives in the past. This may have been at an unconscious as well as a conscious level. Suzie recognised that the final trigger was the socks – a conscious reminder of the inevitability and unpredictability of death, even in her own family. She may have been unconsciously refusing to acknowledge this.

Suzie's experience was affected by the parallels she drew with her own family life and her difficulties in coping with issues related to death and dying. Her reactions and feelings of being out of her depth are common in such situations.

Long after it had happened to her, Salvage (2006:26) described how she remembered with 'a shudder patients who I felt I had failed'. She had a mixture of feelings of anger and grief about a teenage girl who had suffered brain damage during a routine operation and later on was able to see that these feelings were tangled up with her grief for her brother, who had died at the same age. She said: 'At the time I had no way of understanding this. We were offered no support or framework within which to express and explore the emotional and personal meanings of our work' (Salvage, 2006:23). Because of this and of feeling undervalued, overworked and stressed, Salvage described how hard she felt it was to 'dig deep and find caring reserves', leading to what she described as 'compassion fatigue'.

'Compassion fatigue' is sometimes described as 'burn-out'. It is significant not only because of its effect on individual nurses themselves but because it has also been linked with lower patient satisfaction levels (Vahey et al., 2004). It can result in feelings of guilt and failure, loss of motivation, negativism, irritability, tiredness and increased sickness rates. It is associated with emotional 'overload' and the nature of individual resilience to stressful situations but has also been attributed to organisational stressors in the workplace, including heavy workloads and inadequate staffing levels. It can be the result of general feelings of being undervalued or overwhelming demands leading to low morale. It can occur after specific traumatic events but can also happen in staff feeling generally disillusioned by their work experience. It is significant for carers too who, perhaps coping with a loved one day after day, may feel exhausted both physically and emotionally, unsupported and undervalued. Knowledge of the effects of compassion fatigue highlights the importance of recognising the significance of learning about our own emotions (and those of service users and their carers) and of ways of managing them.

Nowadays there are more opportunities for student nurses to discuss their feelings with a mentor, tutor or other colleagues and sometimes through undertaking reflective exercises and assignments. However, reflective assignments can be a response to what is seen to be required academically. Students or qualified staff on courses may not want to, or perceive that it is appropriate to, disclose personal details in writing at such a public level. We need other ways as well for cathartic release and the unpicking of emotions, since we all need help sometimes to make sense of emotional responses which can overwhelm or preoccupy us. Compassion extends to caring for ourselves and our colleagues and noticing the effects of strong emotional experiences. It is often over an informal cup of coffee, in a safe environment, that these experiences are most usefully shared. Emotions should not be perceived as a weakness but part of what makes us who we are.

McCreight (2005) confirmed this, indicating that emotion should be seen as a resource rather than a weakness or deficit. When studying nurses and midwives who were helping women who had experienced miscarriage or stillbirth, she found that they suffered grief and fear when dealing with the loss of a baby – some found it difficult to cope with the emotional distress. However, through analysing their personal feelings (she described this as emotional work), they were able to manage their emotions. McCreight concluded that understanding the meaning of those emotions helped them to develop their professional understanding.

Meeting regularly with colleagues to talk over dilemmas and challenges in practice has been seen as beneficial. Schwarz Centre Rounds began in the USA and are now spreading to the UK. At these, multidisciplinary team members meet monthly to gain insight and support from colleagues (Firth-Cozens and Cornwell, 2009). Graham *et al.* (2005) described how a group of nurses were helped to uncover painful memories of caring for dying patients through reflection. They described the 'mutual suffering' nurses engaged in as a result of feelings of failure and the non-exposure of emotions. The sharing of these feelings through a reflective workshop helped them to conceptualise and articulate their nursing practice. 'The participants found that mutual suffering is a transformational process, leading to professional confusion and personal crisis but it also involves new beginnings and clarification of values and beliefs' (Graham *et al.*, 2005:283). This is an example of how group discussion can help overcome guilt feelings and clarify emotional responses within professional roles and parameters.

Time to think back

We have discussed the important part that emotions play in our practice and how emotional labour may be as demanding as physical labour. Ask yourself the following:

+ Have you been underestimating the extent to which your emotions can both help and develop your understanding of practice?
+ Have you been using theoretical perspectives to help inform your practice and increase your awareness about emotional knowledge? In trying to make sense of a harrowing event, you may have noticed that the student who described her interactions with a young man who had been stabbed used ideas from a variety of sources to help her to recognise and articulate her experience. You may also find it helpful to reflect on emotional 'triggers' in your own practice.
+ Have you found that certain sights, sounds or perhaps even smells have evoked in you an emotional response?
+ Can you think of ways in which reflecting on emotional responses might be facilitated perhaps within mentorship, preceptorship or clinical supervision?
+ Reflecting on all this will help you to understand how important your emotions are in your practice.

Coping with difficult situations

As we have seen, we may find that caring for some people makes other kinds of emotional demands on us. It is natural to acknowledge feelings of anger, fear and even disgust at some of the things we may come across. As we saw in Chapter 3 in our discussion of anti-discriminatory practice, we have to be careful that we recognise these feelings and attitudes in ourselves so that we are able to 'manage' them and prevent them from interfering with the care we provide. The next story, told to us by Petra, a student nurse, illustrates this.

Case Study 4.7

'I was looking after Marge, a patient on an elderly mental infirm (EMI) unit. She was very difficult to nurse as she was extremely aggressive and abusive. It took a lot of time and patience to talk to her. Because of this I often felt that Marge was mainly left to be looked after by the students as the staff nurses did not have enough time.

One day I spent a great deal of time with her, helping her to wash and dress. I sat for about 20 minutes persuading her to take her medication. Every half hour she was doubly incontinent and needed to be cleansed and changed. Her dressing gown was soiled and she didn't have another one. She started to shout at me to fetch her dressing gown for her. No matter how many times I pleasantly and firmly told her that the dressing gown she could see was not hers, but the lady's in the next bed, she continued to yell. She then shouted "You're a lazy bitch, I wish you would all f–off and leave me."

I felt very annoyed and upset at this, but mainly disheartened because of all the time and effort I had put into giving her care even though I knew she couldn't really help it . . .'

Petra's story illustrates the mixture of emotions we might feel when we care for others. At one level she understands both Marge's predicament and her anger but she needs to feel her efforts are being recognised (the need for reciprocity as we discussed in Chapter 2). The story also illustrates that it is often demanding and complex care that is undertaken by the least experienced! It is important to remember that health-care support workers often undertake complex and emotionally draining tasks and for the need to recognise this and enable them also to have the opportunity to talk through their emotions.

As we have said previously, an important part of our professional development is learning how to labour with and manage our emotions, and Petra is beginning to do that. This does not mean ignoring or rejecting her feelings but making an open and honest assessment of what they mean and how they might affect her practice. If we do not do this and are overcome by our emotions, we will feel let down when everything is not as perfect as we would like it to be and we will feel guilty about things we may not be able to do anything about. Conversely, by ignoring them we may disregard and dehumanise people and practise in a routine, unfeeling way in an effort to protect ourselves.

A study by Smith (2003) reveals that many students have some difficulty in disentangling what they see as 'personal emotions' from those expected of a 'professional' but see resolving this as an important part of their professional development. She cites a number of incidents that help demonstrate this, including the following episode written by a third-year student.

'I had to act professionally in this situation because I don't know what I would have felt for this relative who was standing there looking all smart and smug when his wife was practically dying. (According to reports, she had been left for hours before an ambulance was called.) I think that if I hadn't been professional I would have said something wrong – I even felt like hitting him! I was so angry! That poor woman! Looking back on it, I think that it was so wrong of me to have felt that way. I don't think I should have felt so much anger towards him. We are taught not to be judgemental.'

To think about

You can see this third-year student reflects back on her negative feelings and judgement about the patient's husband. She acknowledges she felt very angry with him and then guilty about these feelings, saying 'I think it was so wrong of me . . . We were taught not to be judgemental.'

✦ Have you been 'taught' not to be judgemental? What does this mean for you?
✦ How do you do this on a practical level, for example in a situation such as the above? In what ways can you help health-care support workers in developing non-judgemental care?
✦ Jot down your thoughts and compare them with ours.

Your reflections might be useful as part of your reflective diary or discussions re ethical dimensions of care.

As we discussed in Chapter 1, Smith (1992) described 'surface and deep acting' as part of emotional labour when there is a gap between what you do and what you may feel. This means that through emotional labour we can temporarily suspend our judgement of another's behaviour. By surface acting the student was labouring emotionally and acting at a 'surface level'. The student notes she was able to be professional and did not say anything 'wrong' to the husband – even though she 'even felt like hitting him' at one point.

This was positive in that she did not overtly express her feelings towards the husband of the patient, but as you are probably aware, non-verbal communication often 'leaks through' in our posture, eye contact and so on. She was able to temporarily suspend her judgemental attitude to some degree by this surface acting. We can also change the way we feel by re-arranging our thoughts. Labouring emotionally by 'deep acting' might have helped her, for example, when she felt anger and guilt. The student could have accepted that it is a normal everyday occurrence for us all to make judgements of value and worth about the world and the people in it – this comes from our own frame of reference, past experiences, influenced by our culture, peers, families, education and so on. She might then have acknowledged that she did not know the world of this relative. We therefore need to be very conscious of our feelings towards others and be aware of our prejudices and biases.

Rogers's (1961) description of 'unconditional positive regard' is helpful in this – it is an attitude of mind that makes us positive towards the people we work with, regardless of how we feel about them. Thompson (2002:146) sums this up well. 'This does not mean that we have to like everyone we work with, or that we are "not allowed" to have negative feelings, but it does mean that we need to be as effective as possible with all the people we work with, regardless of feelings towards them or what they may have done. Difficult though it may be to be positive towards people we do not like, good practice requires us to overcome these difficulties.' In other words, to be able to act in a professional manner means that we have to be aware of and suspend our judgements, opinions and beliefs about how the world is. If we 'decentre' or move from our own world with its preoccupations and concerns we will be in a better position to assist those who require our help.

The NMC Code (2008) has an expectation for all nurses and midwives to be non-judgemental when providing care. It states the importance of treating people as individuals and respecting their dignity, not discriminating but treating people kindly and considerately, acting as an advocate and helping them to access relevant health and social care, gain information and support. To do this you need to be aware of any negative or discriminatory feelings you might have and ensure that they do not affect the quality of care you provide. Experienced nurses can do a great deal to help student nurses and health-care support workers by role modelling and enabling discussion without feelings of recrimination or blame, but also in stressing professional responsibilities.

The importance of boundaries in care

Learning the boundaries of professional practice is also bound up with the emotions we feel for patients in our care. In our experience, students need a chance to explore situations in order to learn how professional boundaries can protect both patient and nurse.

An incident from a first-year student nurse highlights this. The student had gone to meet a friend at the station when she saw a patient, who she knew was detained under the Mental Health Act and was particularly vulnerable, getting on a train. She was frightened about what might happen to the patient. Her first thoughts were to distance herself from the situation (she even thought about pretending she had not seen the patient trying to board the train) and yet she decided that, although off duty, she had to act in accordance with a caring, patient-oriented philosophy. She attempted to persuade the patient to go for a cup of coffee to gain time and when this was unsuccessful, she then thought about attempting to stop the train leaving by asking help from a member of the railway staff. She was trying to work within the professional NMC Code of Conduct concerning the need to protect the patient from harm but also thought about the need to maintain confidentiality. Eventually, a telephone call back to the hospital ward was effective in ensuring that strategies were put in place by the ward team and the patient returned safely to the hospital ward.

By talking through her fears and concerns at the time, the student was helped not only to consider the positive and the difficulties in her approach but also to consider professional expectations and boundaries. In nursing we engage in very close relationships, some of which, by their very nature, move outside normal social conventions and barriers, for example in the kind of intimate care we give, or psychological support we provide based on confidential information or knowledge. We must always be sure that we act in the patient's interests and also protect ourselves from the likelihood of misunderstandings. You need to be sure you read and understand any guidance given to staff in your area of practice. You will also find the NMC Code of Conduct (2008) a helpful guide. The student, in alerting the ward team to the possible dangers the patient was in, could be judged to have done what could reasonably be expected in this emergency situation.The need for care to be built on a culture of humane values, service and hospitality is highlighted by MIND (2011), particularly for those who are in hospital against their will. The report draws on the experiences of service users and stresses the importance of organisational commitment and a rethinking of 'professional boundaries' so that staff can interact naturally with the people they are caring for without losing their professionalism (page 6) . The report goes on to recommend to staff teams that they 'share something of yourself in interactions with people using your service - not all your problems but enough to engage on a humane level' (page 43). Could it be that in the drive for keeping within the boundaries of professionalism, nurses have lost something of the natural warmth and humanity that sharing experiences can bring?

Learning to keep a balance

Some of us, finding ourselves in a similar situation to the student at the railway station, might have distanced ourselves from the event. This is a form of detachment that may mean we are actually holding back in order to protect ourselves. This may be a good thing in that we seem to have only a finite set of resources of energy upon which to draw. Part of our emotional labour may be concerned with maintaining a balance of being close, friendly, warm and approachable while still maintaining professional distance. Being overfamiliar or too remote are both unacceptable.

However, it has been argued that sometimes the 'detached' position may not necessarily be a 'wrong place' to be, in that it may also, paradoxically, include a state of readiness for action. As Goleman (1998) notes, those who have the ability to 'keep cool' are admired throughout the world. There are benefits to be gained from those who appear to 'stay collected' when there is an emergency, and/or there is distress or panic. Those who do this can bring a comforting sense of control to the situation. This is especially so if the situation requires immediate and concentrated actions, perhaps to save a life or reduce aggression. Being able to be objective in such situations is an essential part of professional development and also denotes a caring approach.

However, some situations may cause particular distress. It is not uncommon for nurses to sometimes be on the receiving end of verbal abuse and physical violence. It has been recognised that the public should not expect health and social care workers to tolerate violence, bullying and aggression and the Department of Health launched a zero tolerance campaign tackling violence against staff in the NHS (Department of Health, 1999). The NHS Lone Worker Service was set up in 2009 with the objective of providing an accessible, all-encompassing and affordable solution for NHS lone-working staff. This system provides members of staff with a service that they can use to signal discreetly for assistance from the emergency services should they feel vulnerable or distressed when working alone, for example in community care ((NHS Business Services Authority, 2010).

In 2010-11, there was a small increase in reported physical assaults against NHS staff in England: 57,830 compared with 56,718 in 2009-10 (NHS Business Services Authority, 2011). Many of the assaults against NHS staff involve medical factors, such as mental health issues, learning difficulties or conditions such as dementia, and accounted for 69% of that year's assaults. Whilst there has been a rise in criminal prosecutions these are not seen as appropriate if due to medical factors. That may in some part explain why the research showed that in spite of increased awareness, various safeguards and initiatives (e.g. annual CQC staff survey collating figures on assaults and abuse against staff, implementation of a national syllabus for conflict resolution training aimed at all front-line NHS staff) the non-reporting of incidents of both verbal and physical abuse is still an issue. Staff who did not report such incidents gave as the main reason that they were used to it and saw it as 'part of the job'.

Beech and Leather (2003) note the importance of implementing and evaluating student nurse training related to this important aspect. It is also essential for trained staff so that abuse is not seen as an inevitable part of the job. The development of skills, debriefing and shared, supportive critical evaluation of responses and interventions will come some way in overcoming feelings of low morale and low self-esteem that may occur as a result of such occurrences. Nurses are ordinary people who, because of the challenging nature of their work, have to develop a range of coping skills in difficult situations and also antidotes to ameliorate negative behaviour arising from our distress. We have to learn to help each other to be objective, alter our mindset and work against our unhelpful responses so we can learn to educate our emotions and behaviours. Support within the work team for anyone who has experienced such problems is essential, creating an open and caring environment for staff as well as service users. Only then will a culture of compassionate care be possible.

Other situations can upset our emotional balance. A certain 'state of readiness' is key if we are to demonstrate our willingness to deal with situations if and when they arise. Charlie wrote the next incident when she was a staff nurse new to a ward that specialised in vascular surgery. In fact Charlie told us that she was very cross with herself about what happened in this incident because her view of patient care 'has always been humanistic and we as nurses cannot afford to work on automatic pilot'. Read Charlie's story and before you read our explanation which follows, consider these points:

+ Why did Charlie feel guilty and angry with herself?

+ What does the story tell us about 'being in a state of readiness'?

+ What does it tell us about the importance of non-verbal communication?

+ What prompted Bella's progression in the healing process?

Case Study 4.8

'I was working in the acute surgical area, on a late shift. In the afternoon the staffing levels were adequate as there was a reduced operating theatre list. This allowed more time than usual for patient care. The patient was one of 15 on my team. Bella had had a left, above-knee amputation due to peripheral vascular disease. The amputation was the second for Bella, who had needed the same surgery performed on her right leg two years previously. Bella was quite aware that this recent surgery was needed and stated prior to theatre that she was amazed that the second operation had not been performed at an earlier date. For a long time she had suffered from infected ulceration of her left leg and had experienced terrible pain. This had been poorly controlled by medication.

On this particular afternoon, the bandage on her wound site was to be reduced and observed by nursing staff. This was to check that the incision site was healing. As I reduced the bandages, I felt quite relaxed. Bella had experienced an amputation before; therefore I assumed that this would help her cope much better with the recent operation. However, unexpectedly, just as I was removing the tail end of the dressing, Bella burst into tears and started to wail. She declared herself to be an outcast and that she could not bear her present image. She held her hands over her face. My "gut feeling" told me I needed to be close to Bella. I found myself "entering her space" as I lowered my position so that our heights were equal. I met Bella at face level. I sat by her side so that she would know I had time and to be close enough for me to touch her hand as needed.

As we sat, Bella's wails became gentle weeps. I felt the need to be even closer, so I moved my hand from my lap and held her hand. After this I took my hand from her hold and placed it gently on the site of her limb that had been recently removed.

Bella stopped crying immediately and there was a short silence. She looked at me initially with curiosity, perhaps shock, then said calmly in a loud voice, "I am still me, aren't I, Charlie?"

Bella smiled and when she did this I smiled and said, "You will always be you, Bella." After this incident occurred Bella slowly began to resume her usual behaviour. At further wound reviews she never again experienced such upset. She took positive interest in her physiotherapy and rehabilitation programme. I strongly believe that touching her leg after surgery, observing the wound incision and acknowledging the loss of her limb assisted her to come to terms with her altered body image.

Although I was pleased with Bella's progress, knowing that I had helped her, I felt torn and disturbed for days and weeks after the incident had occurred. How could I have assumed that this patient could cope better with that experience because it was not the first? She had lost her remaining leg! I felt frustrated at myself, I had honestly believed that Bella would "know how" this surgery would affect her appearance. I now felt inconsiderate in my initial assumptions. This has taught me that empathy is so very important.'

Compare your considerations with ours

Charlie felt angry with herself and guilty because she thought she ought to have anticipated that Bella would be distraught at losing her second limb through surgical amputation. Charlie detached herself from her focus on the task of wound dressing and recognised Bella's distress. Although taken by surprise, her state of readiness, due in part to her belief in the importance of humanistic care, meant that she was able and willing to disengage from being on 'automatic pilot' and respond to Bella effectively.

The importance of non-verbal communication and the sound and sight of Bella's clear distress signals prompted Charlie's action. She reacted by what she called 'entering into her space', moving her position so that she was at the same level and close to Bella, by using touch (particularly of the affected limb) as a means of reassurance, acknowledgement and comfort.

The interaction between Bella and Charlie helped to progress the healing process. After the therapeutic touch, Bella's 'wails became gentle weeps' and she was suddenly able to step back from her emotions and remembered her own uniqueness. She asked the rhetorical question 'I am still me, aren't I, Charlie?' She already knew the answer because Charlie had acknowledged her as a person. Her self-identity was re-established and this had a positive effect on the way she was able to engage in her physical rehabilitation. Nurses are engaged in work like this in all areas of nursing. They may be helping people who are suffering from altered self-image related to disfigurement from burns or other accidental injury, strokes, surgery or those with mental illness or learning disability.

You may be surprised in Charlie's story at how much effect a seemingly simple interaction can have. As we have found in earlier chapters, this kind of work is hidden and often under-valued even by ourselves. Considered analysis and critical reflection help us to uncover it. Through discussion and support, Charlie was able to see that being new to the ward had a bearing on her being unable to anticipate Bella's grief. The reflective process also helped her to become more self-aware and acknowledge the contribution she made to Bella's care. Otherwise she may have carried these guilt feelings around with her for a long period. She now better understands the need to be gentle with herself and learn from her emotions. She passes this message on to you:

'I hope that other nurses like me realise that it is acceptable to experience guilt, but to know that it also has a place. It is a major move forward for me within my clinical prac-tice to identify and understand guilt more each day. Even though I remain quite critical of myself in clinical practice and find self-praise a difficult task, I hope in time that this will change. Since my experience of sharing and completing the reflective process I feel I have been able to combine personal and professionalism more than ever before. There are still more challenges to be completed in observing the 'self' further to improve my clinical practice. The more nurses experience these situations, the more they can identify with the uniqueness of patients such as Bella, but without forgetting their own being.'

Linking theory and practice

We can see how reflection helps us to uncover important and valuable aspects of nursing. Some might say it teaches us about what care is really all about. It helps us to identify the range of caring skills that help people like Bella and influence their progress. You may have thought of a variety of perspectives that would help shed light on Charlie and Bella's story, such as theories and information about empathy, body image, self-identity and its influence on rehabilitation, non-verbal communication and preparation for surgery. Theories and the evidence base for practice can be wide-ranging and varied – this is what makes nursing so interesting and complex. We thought it might also be useful to carry the discussion a little further.

A significant moment in the story occurred when Bella observed herself and wondered if she was still the same person as she was before the second amputation. Charlie also asked herself questions about her own ability and this led to feelings of anger and guilt that would have affected her self-esteem and therefore self-image. A positive outcome was that she eventually saw her emotional world as a useful focus for learning about herself. Griffin and Tyrrell (2003) claim that we all have an 'observing self' and that this is probably the most significant difference between human beings and the rest of the animal kingdom. They suggest that nature has supplied us with this as a therapeutic restorative–just as both Bella and Charlie found. Discussing the application of their view to therapeutic work, they suggest that 'This is because the observing self is a more fun-damental part of us than even our thinking and feeling selves. It is our awareness that everything else feeds into. A person can lose arms, legs, sight, hearing and yet still have that sense of "I am", and being a centre of experience of reality – "I am aware" . . . All good therapists have the skill to help the client step back into their observing self (even if they don't call it by that name) to identify patterns of conditioning that need to change' (Griffin and Tyrrell, 2003:87).

The story of Charlie and Bella helps show us that if we have warmth, regard, certain understandings and skills, we can help to disengage others and ourselves from emotional, dazed-like states. Our observing self can help us gain a more objective/neutral/unbiased view of our world. This state or way of being is potentially therapeutic as a conscious, logical mind can better objectively check out feelings. In this frame of mind it is possible to question, to scrutinise the situation at hand and to solve problems in more creative ways. In summary, this will help us visualise and plan ways of providing better care.

Effective communication often involves the use of high-level skills that need to be recognised, made explicit and analysed. As practice provides many opportunities for application and development of these skills, their importance should not be overlooked in role modelling and mentoring. An example of this is in what we can gain by analysing the interaction between Bella and Charlie. Goleman (1998:136-137) comments that when we start to connect or communicate with each other we begin 'to fall into a subtle dance of rhythmic harmony'. Movements, postures, vocal pitch, rate of speaking, and even the length of pauses between one person speaking and the other's response, become synchronised. Indeed, in the latter part of the incident, we see Bella taking some control over this synchronisation process. It is as if Bella returns Charlie's understanding and compassionate care by smiling at her, a tribute or thank you to Charlie, and Charlie smiled back – in a subtle dance of harmony. As Goleman (1998:167) asserts, 'Smiling is the most contagious emotional signal of all, having an almost irresistible power to make other people smile in return.'

The work of Rogers (1961) also helps us better understand the abilities and skills associated with empathy. These competencies are about being able to enter the client's world and help them and also being able to get out of the situation without being scathed – that is without being injured or traumatised. Reflection can help us to do this. On a similar note, Goleman (1998:317) argues that we have emotional intelligence that includes 'the ability to recognise our own feelings as well as those of others, for motivating ourselves, and for managing emotions well in ourselves and in our relationships'. If we are to work together effectively as a team, we also have a responsibility to colleagues in helping them to cope with emotional situations.

Helping colleagues to cope

If you are a student, you probably get a great deal of help from other students who share similar fears and concerns to yours. A third-year student told us how she observed a way in which some qualified staff helped each other.

Case Study 4.9

'I was thinking the other day about the ways we survive in nursing and saw more clearly that detaching from all of the emotional baggage is not all that bad. I thought about some of the theories I knew from the literature, such is Pam Smith's research on the emotional labour of nursing and also the "hot action", as Eraut describes aspects of our work when we are so busy we can hardly think straight. I reflected on my own beliefs that we have to learn to detach as a way of protecting ourselves; otherwise we can find ourselves in some sort of "burn-out" position.

I started to see that nurses do "detach" themselves in various ways from it all, otherwise it gets too much. I know that we need to be careful about doing this, because it is so easy to start seeing patients and relatives as less than people and that can be so dangerous. On the other hand, we do need to look after ourselves and I think that this might be an almost 'unseen feature' of our work.

For example, on our ward recently, Wendy, the staff nurse, said to the ward sister, "If you don't mind, I won't go into that cubicle today as I have got a bit of a cold." The sister agreed with Wendy straight away, saying it was fine and that Wendy looked a 'bit under the weather today'. I honestly do not think that Wendy had a cold. She had been caring for a baby who had died the previous day and wanted to keep her distance from any more emotional stuff until she felt strong again and ready to face a new challenge.

I believe that the ward sister knew this was the reason Wendy did not want to go into the cubicle. And Wendy knew that this sister saw past the "I have a cold" excuse. But the cold excuse is a shorthand way of saying "I need to be protected".

It is evident from this story that there was a culture of mutual support that is beneficial to all. However, it does seem a pity that sometimes we are unable to voice our feelings but instead use subtle or covert cues that may or may not be picked up. In this case the 'sickness' was used as a means of restoring balance that may in this instance have been useful but if repeated too often could give rise to a pattern of behaviour that is unhelpful for both the individual and colleagues.

If you are a student, you may find there are several people who help a great deal in giving you support in your 'emotional labour'. As well as peers, perhaps you have gained help from a really good mentor, or a personal tutor. Smith and Gray (2001:233) undertook a study of student nurses and found that link tutors (who visited the students in practice) were helpful. They did this not only by liaising with senior clinical staff and mentors on behalf of the students but also in encouraging reflective learning and informal support, often by identifying with student experiences. 'If my student is having a hard time with a really ill patient, it helps if I can link that with the difficulties I have had. That way you feel you actually feel more about it and can relate to the student. It helps to work it through with them and see what to do next.'

Just as we've been able to learn a great deal from nurses' stories throughout this text, so, it would seem, the very act of telling the story helps to clarify significant events. It is also interesting that Smith and Gray found that students and mentors found it easier to talk about good practice than to write about it. Perhaps it is the informality of sharing stories and ideas that makes this a particularly useful strategy and allows us to uncover details we might otherwise have overlooked. The authors concluded that the role of reflection, storytelling and the use of oral accounts are ways of accumulating evidence to demonstrate the content and process of emotional labour in teaching, learning and caring. Mentors and link tutors have a central role in ensuring this occurs. However, this is a two-way process. As a student, how you react to your mentor, tutors and other colleagues will influence your learning experience by, for example, whether you are able and willing to engage in reflective conversations. It is all too easy for qualified nurses to miss out on coffee or meal breaks when too busy whether working in hospital or community venues. We should, however, see these as essential for restorative balance, both physically and emotionally. The opportunity to share experiences with colleagues is not just enjoyable but essential for our well-being.

In later chapters, we will be discussing more about how you might develop your ability to engage in reflective discussions and find ways of increasing your self-awareness and becoming more analytical about your emotional reactions to situations.

Summary

In this chapter, we have explored the emotional world of nursing and have seen the relevance of acknowledging and using our emotions as a resource for developing our caring skills. We have seen how our balance may be disrupted as we work within professional boundaries and personal expectations.

+ We have found that the emotional world of nursing can be demanding but also intensely satisfying.
+ We have seen how nurses, engaged in everyday tasks which bring them close to patients, can help overcome problems related to self-image.
+ We have learned more about the part emotions can play in the way in which nurses see their practice and react to situations, including the way they make judgements and behave.
+ Identification with particular patients and objects can act as triggers and affect our emotional balance.
+ We have seen the importance of using opportunities for reflective learning both for ourselves and for others. This includes gaining knowledge of high-level communication skills and more understanding of boundaries of our professional relationship with service users and their families.

Looking forward

A major focus of care in all aspects of nursing is related to caring for people with long-term health-care needs. Because of this, most of this care now takes place in the community and is likely to increase even further in the future. In the next chapter, we will explore the challenges of developing caring and effective relationships with service users and their carers. These are people with vast experience and we need to capture and utilise this. More care is undertaken by informal carers, perhaps assisted by multi-professional teams. We will use stories from service users, students and qualified nursing staff to help us learn more about the way in which we can develop effective and supportive caring partnerships by pooling our knowledge and resources.

Activity

Look at the caring indicators and use them to explore your own emotional world of practice. You may find them useful to prompt your reflections, either verbally or in a written form. The aim of this activity will be for you to see how knowledge of your emotions will help you to improve your caring skills.

Caring indicators

1. Using emotional labour as a resource for developing caring skills – turning compassion into effective nursing actions

2. Being in a state of readiness for action, 'keeping cool' in stressful situations and restoring emotional balance after an event

3. Recognising 'triggers' in specific events, especially those that undermine our usual coping strategies

4. Developing high-level communication skills using appropriate touch and other non-verbal and verbal communication; avoiding rash and discriminatory judgements

5. Finding ways of coping with or managing upsetting situations and being sensitive to the needs and feelings of other health-care workers, service users and their families

6. Using opportunities that promote a patient's positive self-image

7. Maintaining a balance of emotions, being neither hardened nor overemotional

8. Understanding and keeping within the boundaries of professional practice without losing natural warmth and humanity

9. Creating an open and caring environment to provide a 'culture of compassionate care', e.g. by recognising 'compassion fatigue' in staff or carers, excellent role modelling, passing on tacit practice knowledge

10. Challenging and reporting actions which can lead to dehumanised practice or incidents of abuse or assault on staff

References

Beech, B and Leather, P (2003) Evaluating a management of aggression unit for student nurses. *Journal of Advanced Nursing* **44**, 603–612.

Chambers, C and Ryder, E (2009) *Compassion and caring in nursing*. Oxon: Radcliffe Publishing Ltd.

Department of Health (1999) *NHS zero tolerance campaign tackling violence against staff in the NHS*. London: DoH.

Dizon, A (2007) Health care practitioners in a people-centred care system. In *People Centred health care – technical papers*. Geneva: World Health Organisation Available at: **www.wpro.who.int/NR/rdonlyres/4D90B8CA-0CA549AS-A93C-4CDBC6D91808/0/PCItechPapers20Aug2008.pdf** (last accessed 27/02/ 2012).

Eastbrooks, C and Morse, J (1992) Toward a theory of touch: the touching process and acquiring a touching style, *Journal of Advanced Nursing* **17**, 448–456

Firth-Cozens, J and Cornwell, J (2009) *The Point of Care; enabling compassionate care in acute hospital settings*. London: King's Fund.

Gibson, M and Iwaniec, D (2003) An empirical study into the psychosocial reactions of staff working as helpers to those affected by the aftermath of two traumatic incidents. *British Journal of Social Work* [online] **33**, 851–870. Available at: **www.proquest.umi.com** (last accessed 3 July 2007).

Goleman, D (1998) *Working with Emotional Intelligence*. London: Bloomsbury.

Graham, I, Andrewes, T and Clark, L (2005) Mutual suffering: a nurse's story of caring for the living as they are dying. *International Journal of Nursing Practice* **11**, 277-285.

Griffin, J and Tyrrell, I (2003) *Human Givens: A new approach to emotional health and clear thinking*. Chalvington, UK: HG Publishing.

James, N (1992) Care = organisation + physical labour + emotional labour. *Sociology of Health and Illness* **14**, 488-505.

Mackintosh, C (2006) Caring, the socialisation of pre-registration students nurses, a longitudinal study. *International Journal of Nursing Studies* **55**, 4, 465- 477.

McCreight, B (2005) Perinatal grief and emotional labour: a study of nurses' experience in gynae wards. *International Journal of Nursing Studies* **42**, 439-448.

MIND (2011) *Listening to experience in acute and crisis mental health care*. Available at: **www.mind.org.uk/assets/0001/5921/Listening_to_experience_web.pdf.** last accessed 24/02/12).

NHS Business Services Authority (2010) Violence against NHS frontline staff. Available online at **www.nhsbsa.nhs.uk**. (last accessed 1/03/2112).

NHS Business Services Authority (2011) Criminal sanctions rise for assaults on NHS staff in 2011. Available at: **www.nhsbsa.nhs.uk** (last accessed 1/03/211).

NMC (Nursing and Midwifery Council) (2008) *The Code: Standards of conduct, performance and ethics for nurses and midwives*. London: NMC.

Parkinson, F (1997) *Critical Incident Debriefing: Understanding and dealing with trauma*. London: Souvenir Press.

Phillips, S (1996) Labouring the emotions. *Journal of Advanced Nursing* **24**, 139-143.

Rogers, C (1961) *On Becoming a Person*. London: Constable.

Ronaldson, S (2000) *Spirituality: The Heart of nursing*. Parkville, Vic.: Ausmed Publications.

Salvage, J (2006) It's the action that counts. *Nursing Standard* **20**, 20-23.

Schutz, S, Angove, C and Sharp, P (2004) Assessing and evaluating reflection. In Bulman, C and Schutz, S (eds) *Reflective Practice in Nursing*. Oxford: Blackwell.

Smith, A (2003) Learning about reflection. PhD thesis. Northumbria University, Newcastle upon Tyne.

Smith, A and Russell, J (1991) Using critical incidents in nurse education. *Nurse Education Today* **11**, 284-291.

Smith, P (1992) *The Emotional Labour of Nursing: How nurses care*. London: Macmillan.

Smith, P and Gray, B (2001) Reassessing the concept of emotional labour in student nurse education: the role of link lecturers and mentors in a time of change. *Nurse Education Today* **21**, 230-237.

Strauss, A, Fagerhaugh, S, Suczek, B and Weiner, C (1982) Sentimental work in the technologised hospital. *Sociology of Health and Illness* **4**, 254-277.

Thompson, N (2002) *People Skills*. Basingstoke: Palgrave Macmillan.

Vahey, D, Aiken, L, Sloane, D, Clarke, S and Vargas, D (2004) Nurse burnout and patient satisfaction. *Medical care*, 42,2,57-61.

Chapter 5

Creating caring partnerships with service users and their families

LEARNING OBJECTIVES

By the end of this chapter you should have an understanding of:

1. Creating effective partnerships with carers and those receiving care
2. The challenges of, and opportunities for, sustaining caring approaches within changing care and social contexts
3. The importance of having a blend of caring attitudes, knowledge and competent skills in caring for others
4. The importance of maintaining a continuity of care and engagement in effective multi-professional and multi-agency approaches
5. Ways in which theory can help to us to reflect critically on practice

Introduction

It is easy to forget just how much care is undertaken by 'informal' carers - partners, parents, daughters, sons, friends and neighbours who do so out of love and perhaps a sense of duty. The 2001 Census (Department of Health, 2009) gives us some understanding of this, indicating that there are approximately 5.2 million people in the UK who provide unpaid care for a relative, friend or neighbour and in doing so make a significant contribution to the care provided in the community. The largest group of carers are in the 50+ age range (about a third of these are over 65), and over a million spend 50 hours a week or more on providing care.

The increase in the number of people requiring help is related to greater life expectancy and medical success in treating people, including children, with chronic illnesses. There has also been a decrease in the number of hospitals and institutions for people with long-term needs. Decisions concerning health, education and social care are made by each devolved government in the UK but all have responded to public pressure to recognise the value of carers and provide better support. The National Carers Strategy was published in June 2008 (Department of Health, 2008) with the aim that; 'by 2018, carers will be universally recognised and valued as being fundamental to strong families and stable communities . . . Support will be tailored to meet individuals' needs, enabling carers to maintain a balance between their caring responsibilities and a life outside caring, while enabling the person they support to be a full and equal citizen' (pages 9-10).

In England, a follow-up report - the 'Next steps for Carers strategy' (Department of Health 2010:2) - promised to facilitate this, giving more control to carers, with personal budgets provided for everyone eligible by April 2013. Outcomes were identified related to recognition of carers as experts and support to ensure they are enabled to have a life of their own alongside their caring role. More support (including financial) was promised to enable them to stay mentally and physically well. Children and young people who have a caring role are particularly mentioned and promised that 'they will be protected from inappropriate caring and have the support they need to learn, develop and thrive and to enjoy positive childhoods' (page 5).

It would seem, therefore, that at last more attention is being paid to what is often euphemistically called 'informal care', which may be very demanding (Yeandle *et al.*, 2007). However, there is a real challenge to make government pledges a reality. Spencer *et al.* (2011:8) note that 'It is well recognised that carers, while making a major contribution to health and social care in the community, are generally poorly supported. They may suffer significant health problems themselves, and economic hardship, and their voice often goes unheard. Together these circumstances present new challenges for working more effectively with patients, their carers and families.'

It is very important that at this time we as professional carers take this opportunity to work with and support informal carers more effectively. In this chapter we will consider how nurses can help to sustain caring approaches, taking into account changes as the result of an expansion in the nature and amount of community care and the need to provide more help and support to those who give care for most of the time. We will explore the nature of the relationship between professionals, service users and informal carers, and consider the opportunities for, and challenges of, creating effective partnerships. Stories based on experience will continue to help us understand better ways of helping people and how we can use resources and theoretical frameworks to ensure we are caring in our approaches.

Living with a member of the family who has dementia

Caring for a relative with dementia may bring with it particular demands that can be emotional, physical, economic and social and that can have an impact over a prolonged period of time. With increased longevity has come a rise in the number of people suffering from Alzheimer's disease and so often the main carers may be older partners with health problems themselves. Feelings such as guilt, frustration, concern, loss of hope and a sense of helplessness may arise for the carer as well as for the person suffering from dementia, who may also experience loss of self-identity and self-esteem. This is more likely if the carer is under a great deal of stress and is unable to cope with situations that may arise.

Consider the following account written by a student nurse and think about the main issues that need to be considered. Compare your responses with ours.

Case Study 5.1

'We were asked to visit Harriet who had been discharged from hospital following a chest infection but had also been diagnosed with Alzheimer's disease. She lived with her daughter Rosie and her family. Rosie met us at the door and was close to tears. "I feel I'm at the end of my tether," she said. "I've been up half the night. At 3 a.m. I heard Mum – she had turned the radio on full blast and was sweeping the stairs. I tried to reason with her – and told her that it was the middle of the night – she became very stubborn – told me that it was the morning and she had to make an early start and get the work done. Eventually I persuaded her to sit down and have a cup of tea and then managed to get her back to bed but I couldn't get to sleep myself as I was worried that she would get up and turn the gas cooker on as she did a night or so ago. She seems much worse since she has been ill with the chest infection. My sister comes in to help as I go out to work and we really wanted to be able to look after her ourselves but we're finding it very difficult to cope."'

Compare your considerations with ours

More and more people find themselves in this situation, particularly women who are in full- or part-time employment but trying to do a 'juggling act' by also looking after relatives who need care. Rosie needs help if she is to continue to be able to care for her mother. The immediate need is to respond empathetically to her distress and talk through strategies to get practical help.

You may have wondered what Harriet thought about all this and the level at which she might be functioning or be helped to function. Despite any cognitive impairment she might have, it is important to remember that a sense of self can be retained even at the very end stages of dementia. This has been described by Kitwood (1997) as a sense of personhood which is underpinned by feelings of personal worth, a sense of agency (which means that he or she can still make things happen), social confidence and acceptability, and hope. Harriet should be given an opportunity to participate in decisions and arrangements made about her care if she is able. Aggarwal et al. (2003:188) highlight ways that will help us to access the views and feelings of those with dementia, including 'adapting to their pace and timescale, taking account of environmental factors and studying non-verbal communication'. This will help not only Harriet but also Rosie and the rest of the family. Nurses themselves have identified a lack of knowledge concerning how to care for people with dementia (Francis, 2010). Consequently, there is a drive to provide more training so that health and social care staff may understand the needs of individuals and their carers and so that interventions occur before breaking point as experienced by Rosie (Skills for care, Skills for Health, Department of Health 2011). The Alzheimer's Society have produced a 'This is me' leaflet which is available online (**www.Alzheimers.org.uk**) to give to staff when a person with dementia goes into hospital. It provides information about a person's individual preferences, likes and dislikes.

You may also have questioned the quality of the discharge planning. There may have been pressure on bed occupancy within the hospital so Harriet may have been discharged as soon as her acute medical condition (chest infection) improved, with very little thought or planning into how the condition and hospitalisation might have had an impact on her overall level of functioning. More communication between the hospital and community team as well as a full assessment of her functioning and well-being would have helped. Input from a dementia specialist nurse, if the hospital had one, would also have helped.

You might also have considered the blurring of the boundaries between health and social care. Who will take responsibility to help Harriet and Rosie? Multi-agency work is a key factor here and consideration has to be given to determine which professional colleagues and agencies will be able to help best in assessing, planning and implementing a care package. A social work referral is essential if this has not yet occurred. Caring in this case might be helping Rosie to explore the resources available to her. There are numerous websites that are useful for this, including the Department of Health website on **www.direct.gov.uk**, or carers' websites such as **www.carersuk.org** or **www.alzheimers.org.uk** which will give Rosie (and you) information on carers' rights, financial support and national and local support groups.

Linking theory and practice

As Rosie feels she is at 'the end of her tether' she needs as much help as possible if she is to be able to continue to care for her mother. Marion Witton (2003), a nurse herself, provided a moving account of her own family's experiences of coping with her mother who was diagnosed as suffering from Alzheimer's disease. She suggests that there is a time when a family is able to recognise this. She described the effect on the family of many distressing changes in her mother, who became depressed and anxious, lost her memory, complained a lot, became self-absorbed, having no interest in anyone but herself, and dependent on her husband, not letting him out of her sight. Marion wrote: 'It is never easy to have to accept "outside" help in the form of services. The emotions of dealing with the deterioration of a loved one and the feeling of "failure" to do everything yourself are hard to admit' (2003:15). A caring nurse will recognise this and, working in partnership with families and as a member of a supportive team, will help a family to cope. In Marion's case, her family was helped to turn a distressing situation into a manageable one. She explained this as follows. 'Nothing was imposed. The many people involved through the health-care and the voluntary sectors were efficient yet understanding and caring. The legislation and ethos of community care worked for us in that what was given was not just to the patient but to the whole family' (2003:15).

Marion's experience reflects positive work that is taking place to support families in caring ways. As mentioned in earlier chapters, a significant amount of care, particularly within the community, is still provided by women, although, with the changing role of women in society with more engaged in full-time work and also interested in career advancement, the balance may be changing (Morrison and Bennett, 2006). Nevertheless, there is still an expectation that a woman will take on responsibility for the caring role and this usually falls to a daughter, although if a son is the nearest or only next of kin, it may well be a daughter-in-law. The expectation of caring as 'women's work' may account for it being seen as 'natural', 'their duty' and 'unskilled'. As we have seen, however, it may not be an easy or a short-term task. Taking responsibility for the care of another person, of whatever age group, may last a number of years and may be very challenging. In addition, many middle-aged women may now not only find themselves responsible for the care of an older relative but also caring for preschool grandchildren. Professionals, therefore, have to work closely with carers and draw on multi-professional and voluntary resources if they are to support families within the community and help maintain the quality of life for carers as well as those being cared for.

There may be other difficulties in that if family members caring for an older person continue working, they may find that their employer's 'family-friendly' policies and practices are not designed to address the needs of staff members who care for older and disabled adults, as they are more likely to be geared towards the needs of working parents of young children, although even this may be difficult.

To think about

+ Who does the caring in your family?
+ What does this entail?
+ What are the implications in terms of possible stresses, but also benefits?

You may have found that, in your family, although caring is shared amongst different members and that although more men are now taking on a caring role, many women continue to take a major role in this, even if they are in paid employment. Caring for someone usually involves a mixture of physical, emotional and social tasks. You may have highlighted tasks such as personal help with washing, shopping, cleaning, cooking or providing meals, paying bills, taking someone out, keeping them company, comforting and ensuring they are safe and protected. This is a way of demonstrating love or regard for a person, or could be undertaken out of a sense of duty. Rewards from care giving include seeing others benefiting from the care we provide and helping to create an environment where others can develop and/or cope with difficult situations. Carers may then feel positive about themselves as they are developing or continuing satisfying relationships. This is all part of the process of giving and receiving in care, as discussed in Chapter 2.

Caring can be hard work, and requires complex and wide-ranging skills. It can be emotionally very demanding, restrict social opportunities for carers and cause stress and worry. Phillips *et al.* (2002) studied the impact on women working as formal carers (in health and social care) but who also had responsibilities as informal carers (suggesting perhaps that being a nurse or a social worker might mean that other members of the family delegate the responsibility of care to them). These authors found that the majority of the women did not allow their caring responsibilities to have an impact on their work, which sometimes acted as a buffer and was important for the women carers in terms of self-esteem and identity. However, the increasing demands on them were more likely to affect their family life and their own health, particularly in terms of stress and tiredness.

Support on the practical and emotional level, including supportive friends, colleagues and managers (who helped keep things in perspective), assisted them in being able to juggle the responsibilities of many competing demands but they also needed key organisational skills, e.g. in making out rotas. Phillips *et al.* found that seemingly straightforward strategies helped the women to cope and to 'avoid care overload'. Such strategies included being able to talk over problems with someone else, being able to draw not only on their own expertise but also on the experience they were building up, seeing the funny side of a situation and maintaining their outside interests. This study has important lessons for us in terms of what we may be called upon to do in both our personal and our professional lives and what is helpful to enable carers to continue to care in the community. As men take on more of such responsibilities, we also need to recognise that needs, particularly those of older men giving care, are complex and may be gender specific (Witucki-Brown *et al.*, 2007). They may, for example, be reluctant to ask for help or have feelings of inadequacy if they do so.

In Chapter 2 we described the study by Brouwer *et al.* (2005), who found that, instead of seeing it as a burden, many informal care givers reported positive benefits from providing care to their loved one and that on average their happiness levels would decline if this care was handed over to someone else. It is in the interest of everyone, therefore, to work effectively in partnership with carers such as Rosie to help maintain the positive benefits of providing care.

Creating caring partnerships with carers

As professionals we must ensure that we work with families as equal partners. If professionals disregard what may be seen as something as straightforward and basic as conventional good manners, the partnership will seem one-sided and disrespectful. You can see evidence of this in Gudrun's story.

Case Study 5.2

'We were due to have a meeting at the family home with a social worker and the specialist health visitor; an educational officer was also invited to attend.

Firstly, the health visitor could not remember what time the meeting was to be held so she called at ten minutes past eight in the morning. My husband let her in and she told him, "I am just going to wait until the meeting starts." The meeting was actually at 9.30 a.m. So, basically she sat in the middle of our living room. It was the usual total morning chaos in our house (with people running around half dressed and trying to get the others out to school and work).

The problem for me was that she seemed to have disregarded the fact that we were a family and she was treating us as a "case". The fact that this was in our home seemed to be totally irrelevant to her and she did not value our privacy and show us respect.

We are not a "disabled project" or a "disabled family"; we are a family who happens to have a disabled child.'

You can see the way Gudrun has used particular language to describe the differences between how she views her situation and how she thinks the health visitor viewed her family. Simply by the health visitor not arriving at a more appropriate time or even apologising, Gudrun feels that the needs and privacy of her family have not been appreciated and respected. Privacy is an important aspect and note how Gudrun links it with showing respect. Privacy is often related to physical care or information sharing, which are important aspects but it is also necessary to remember that families of vulnerable children or adults should be treated with respect and protected from unwarranted interference. Gudrun also thought her problems would be helped if professionals worked together as a team, sharing information and assessing the whole family's needs.

In response to the UK government's personalisation agenda, a report from the Princess Royal Trust and Crossroads for Caring (2009) noted that carers have had to fight over many years to gain recognition as 'partners in care', and too often they thought that they were still left with all of the responsibility but none of the support for or acknowledgement of the role they perform. There is a real challenge for nurses to work together with other agencies in active partnerships so that carers feel that services are 'on their side' (DOH, 2009:5). Gudrun emphasised this aspect:

Case Study 5.3

'We want a joined-up approach to our care; I get sick of repeating the same information to all of the professionals who visit us. There should be one person who can take the information and share it. I know they need profession-specific details, but there is a central core of information that they all want! For example, Billy has a physiotherapist, an occupational therapist, a paediatrician, a speech therapist, a dietitian, a peripatetic educationalist for the visually impaired and he receives "formal care" during the day when I am at work (this carer has a qualification in nursery nursing and has looked after Billy since he was two).

I think this is important for nurses to consider in that they may play a central role in the assessment and organisation of care needs for the child and family. The nurse really can "get it all together" for the family if they do their job properly. For us this would include information about how Billy's younger sister is affected by this. All of her life it has been "Hang on till we do this for Billy and that for Billy." Sometimes it feels like it is me against the system and it should not be like that; the nurse would help me with the advocacy required to get what Billy needs. This is what I think the government means by a joined-up approach. This is not what happens now, irrespective of what and how professionals are taught at the moment.'

It appears that the government has recognised the importance of supporting informal carers like Gudrun and is listening to what they are saying and the increasing confidence which greater public access to websites and support networks has given carers will ensure that their voices continue to be heard. Nurses have important opportunities to act as advocates for those who may not be able to make themselves heard or understood and also to recognise the expertise of those who may be caring for them. Sasha's story illustrates how problematic this may be.

Case Study 5.4

'My daughter has been ill for many years with bipolar disorder. Her relationship with her husband is difficult at times and when she is ill, he copes by immersing himself in work, so I take over as her main carer and also of her young family. However, I find it really aggravating that I have to really fight to get professionals to listen to me about changes in her behaviour which I know will lead to problems. I think they regard me as an interfering mother. In the past, the situation has had to reach a crisis point and she has had to be "sectioned" before she gets the care she requires.'

Relationships within families are complex and varied and it would seem that Sasha's story illustrates the importance of getting to know the whole family situation so that individuals taking caring roles can be best supported. If this is so, they in turn will provide the best support for the person needing medical help or long-term monitoring. In this case both the husband and Sasha would have benefited by their views being sought out and acknowledged by health professionals and also by the adoption of an open and honest approach to any decisions made about the girl's care. Jenkins, a member of the Standing Commission on Carers (Department of Health, 2009), highlights this, indicating that

'Carers often have a deep insight into the condition of the person they are caring for, especially for a fluctuating condition such as a mental illness. They need to be treated by professionals as "Partners in Care". Too often patient confidentiality is used as a reason for excluding carers, leading to poorer outcomes for all and sadly on occasions putting the person and their carers at risk.' (page 10)

As the nature of care work changes, the skills needed to help others fulfil a caring role change too. If followed through effectively, government policies can be extremely helpful in supporting and guiding carers, but as we know, many people need help to avail themselves of the opportunities present and may still need one-to-one advice from a health or social care professional. Nurses are often in an excellent position to provide this and strong cases have to be made for the retention of specialist nurses who can provide expert advice and guidance to colleagues as well as patients and carers on best approaches to care. A more personalised approach to care also requires nurses to work more closely with colleagues in other disciplines so that effective seamless, inter-agency care is provided.

The importance of continuity of care for carers

Sometimes thoughtless care can undo what has been achieved over a long period of time. Read Luke's account of his father's stay in hospital and consider what problems there were and the benefits which might have been gained from ensuring a better relationship with the relatives.

Case Study 5.5

'Following his severe stroke we worked really hard for three months to help Dad regain continence. He then went into a respite centre to allow my wife and me a long weekend. Just before we left we had a telephone call informing us that Dad had fallen and hurt his back. He was admitted to the local hospital and the consultant told him that he would remain there till we returned home. Dad told her he hadn't passed urine since his admission. Because the consultant knew our concerns about the length of time it had taken to get him continent, she asked the junior doctor to pass a catheter, drain the bladder and remove it.

On return from our weekend, Dad had been moved to another ward. We noticed a very, and I mean very, full catheter drainage bag alongside the bed. I was furious and went to see the nurse in charge. She informed me that the use of a catheter was standard practice and couldn't be taken out until the doctors did their rounds the next day.

The following morning, the registrar agreed to speak to us. In response to my protests that it had taken three months for Dad to regain continence, he said the catheter would be removed. On visiting in the evening Dad was sitting out in a chair. Although the catheter had been removed, he didn't know where the toilets were and was sitting in his sodden trousers. Nothing was recorded in the fluid balance sheets. A care assistant came to help clean and change Dad. When we visited the next day it was apparent that he was regressing. He was sodden again, so I took him to the bathroom to wash and change him. Dad then decided that he wanted to go for a walk and proceeded to walk to the ward exit. "I want to come home," he said. We saw the nurse in charge and explained our concerns. The next morning he was discharged. It took two months for him to regain continence to the level experienced before the re-catheterisation.'

Problems

+ Lack of coordination and continuity in care meant that decisions were not communicated and acted upon, which made Luke feel as if all the care and continence promotion that the family had provided were disregarded.

+ In the second ward, catheterisation appeared to be 'routine' rather than a considered decision based on individual circumstances. Luke felt that hospital staff had taken the easy route. He told us, 'Catheters are easy to pass and do control incontinence, but at what price to the patient and carer?'

Reasons for a better relationship

+ Care did not begin and end with the professional input but was a continuum of care, with the major amount undertaken by Luke and his wife. Their views, and those of their father, should have been taken into account.

+ Luke's father did not feel cared for. He suffered loss of dignity, self-esteem and feelings of powerlessness. It is no wonder he wanted to go home. Once more he had to go through an intensive relearning process. His experience might also affect the way in which he viewed any professional help or hospitalisation in the future. Neither he nor his relatives had trust in the professional care they were receiving.

+ The fact that Luke and his wife needed respite care indicates that they may have found caring for their Dad tiring and at times demanding. If more attempts had been made in promoting continence, the impact of the hospitalisation might have been less stressful.

+ The lack of coordination with, and respect for, relatives may have resulted in long-reaching consequences if they then felt no longer able to cope - having an impact both economically and in terms of a greater need for resources in general.

It becomes increasingly evident that it is essential that nurses work in partnerships with carers whether they are providing care in hospital or community so there is continuity in the quality of that care. There may be many considerations to take into account as increasingly, with demographic changes in society and an ageing population, at times the carer may also be a person who is receiving care themselves or, conversely, the care provider may be a child.

Children as carers

Read Sharon and Roberto's story summarised below and consider what effect you think caring for his mother might have on Roberto in terms of his development and quality of life. Then compare your considerations with ours.

Case Study 5.6

Roberto is 10 years old and lives with his mother, Sharon, who suffers from a bipolar affective disorder. Sharon's illness means that at times she can be overactive and emotionally very 'high' and at other times she is very depressed and finds it difficult to be motivated to do anything, even to get up in the morning. She is embarrassed about her illness and because she feels friends and neighbours would not understand it, and would probably think she is 'not right in the head', she tends to keep herself to herself and socialise very little. There are no other members of the family living close by. Although the medication helps to control her mood swings, she is sometimes unable to undertake the usual activities of living such as cooking, shopping, cleaning etc., and this then falls to Roberto. Sharon feels guilty about her reliance on Roberto and told us, "I've tried my best but I know I ask him to do too much. I try and make sure he is still able to enjoy himself but if I need help, he is the one whom I rely on. He does all sorts of things – he can cook a meal, make a cup of tea, do the shopping and clean up. He cheers me up and makes me laugh when I'm down. He gets me to do things I wouldn't otherwise feel like doing – like taking my medication." Sharon says she is a little wary of professionals. When she has been hospitalised in the past, Roberto received respite care and she is very frightened that he might be taken into care permanently.

Mick is a community psychiatric nurse who became Sharon's key worker. He recognised the close relationship between mother and son and made a point of spending time talking with Roberto to see what he thought about the situation and assess the effect it was having on him. Roberto felt that Mick was looking after both of them.

'He told me I was doing a good job with Mum and told me anything I needed to know about what was happening to her and what I should do in an emergency or if I was worried about anything. Sometimes I get a bit miffed if I can't get out to football practice when Mum needs me at home but most of the time it's OK – we sort things out. Mick got Annie, the social worker, to come and see me and she got me to join the young carers support group at Barnardo's. It's good to talk to other kids in the same boat and we have a laugh!'

Compare your considerations with ours

You may have been concerned about Roberto, wondering about the effects that having so much responsibility might have on his psychological, social and educational development. You may think that he is 'losing his childhood' and the opportunities to enjoy himself with his peers. However, you will have also noticed that Roberto sees positive as well as negative effects. This was helped by having positive feedback from Mick so he felt recognised and appreciated for his efforts. Mick gave Roberto information which helped him to look after his mother better. This is an indication of an equitable and non-patronising partnership.

You might also have considered Sharon's role as a caring mother. The relationship between mother and son is one of closeness and it is therefore one of giving and receiving for both partners – one of mutuality and reciprocity as we saw in Chapter 2. Roberto is still receiving love and interest from his mother, although at times this might be hard for her to show in a physical sense. Looking after the whole family means that Sharon is more likely to able to fulfil her role as a mother.

Mick worked effectively with Annie the social worker so that, through joining a young carers group, there was an opportunity for Roberto to feel he had something in common with other children and could gain support and social benefits.

There is evidence that the number of children caring for parents or siblings has been underestimated. The 2001 UK census identified 175,000 but parents completed the form on behalf of their families and they might not have wanted to admit to being cared for or having problems. However, a survey conducted by the BBC and University of Nottingham in 2010 of more than 4,000 UK school pupils found one in 12 had moderate or high levels of caring responsibility (dressing, washing, bathing) and the authors concluded that there are likely to be four times the number identified in 2001. In addition there are a 'hidden' number of children who regularly provide emotional care. These may not be considered as young carers, but it is likely that many of them are providing support for family members with mental illnesses or addictions to drugs or alcohol.

Using research to gain more knowledge

More knowledge is needed about possible effects on children as carers. Aldridge and Becker (2003) conducted a study of children and young people under 18 years old who were caring for parents with enduring mental health problems. They came up with some interesting find-ings. A prime concern of the parents in the study related to the prognosis of their illness and how this would affect their children. They were concerned that the children lacked support when they were undertaking care and the authors considered that this could become an enduring and stressful aspect of the parents' mental ill health experience and could in turn create further crises for the family. Aldridge and Becker found, however, that whilst mental illness may result in a loss of parenting function or a child having to fulfil a parent-like role, as seems apparent with Sharon and Roberto, it can also cement parent–child relationships. They suggest that there is a need to improve our understanding of children's experience of caring when parents are affected by illness as these relationships are often perceived by professionals in health and social care as negative. Consulting children themselves can uncover positive as well as adverse experiences, e.g. that providing the care themselves reduces some of their anxieties and fears.

> 'Our evidence shows that the damaging effects of children caring for and living with parents with mental health problems are not determined by the mental illness in itself and of itself, but by a range of other factors including isolation and exclusion (from care plans, service interventions, approaches from family and professionals and community misunderstanding and discrimination in particular), as well as by other social determi-nants (including low income, poverty and so on).' (Aldridge and Becker 2003:95)

Children, they claim, may suffer from information deficit (and information should be provided in a way which is age-related) and that 'whole family' approaches should be used so that they are both consulted and can talk to someone they can trust and who understands their needs both as children and as carers. There is evidence from their research that professionals across a range of disciplines felt able and competent to describe the effects on children based on their assumptions and not through close contact with children and their families. Therefore, although there is acknowledgement that some effects on children may be extremely detrimental, there is a call for professionals to use effective assessment and intervention strategies which will give children some degree of choice in undertaking care responsibilities. Whilst Roberto's story reinforces the need for us not to make assumptions about who is able or not able to provide care and to recognise the complexities and variety of care relationships, it is also necessary for ensuring that children who are carers have the opportunity to 'learn, develop and thrive and to enjoy positive childhoods' (DOH 2010:5).

The complexity of caring partnerships

For some families who are struggling to care, there may be many difficulties that complicate the relationship between them and the professionals who try to help them. Susan, a student in placement with the community children's nursing team, told us about problems that arose when working with Ami and her family. Read her story, make a note of the difficulties and then compare your thoughts with ours.

Case Study 5.7

'Ami was born prematurely to Stephanie and Liam, who are a very young mother and father, both still in their teens. Before she had Ami, Stephanie had been "sleeping rough" on the streets and it is believed she probably had taken drugs on a regular basis before and during part of her pregnancy. My mentor said that because Ami had been born early and had cerebral palsy and epilepsy she was kept in the special care baby unit and had to be fed via a nasogastric tube. Stephanie and Liam only stayed for a short time when they visited Ami and the social worker assisted the nurses in arranging a meeting with them to encourage them to get involved with feeding Ami via the tube so she could go home with them. This proved easier said than done as the parents sometimes failed to attend the unit for the teaching sessions and, when they did, it seemed to be a very difficult "task" for them, in part due to Ami's very jerky thrashing arm movements and poor head control. Because of these problems the community children's team was involved prior to and after Ami's discharge from hospital.

When we visited Ami at home we found that both parents were insistent that they were managing very well, "thank you", and adamant that they gave her tube feeds according to the dietitian's plan, although my mentor was concerned because Ami was not putting on weight. Stephanie in particular seemed to be not worried about this, appeared disinterested and did not seem to have bonded with Ami. She got very angry when my mentor asked questions, such as whether they were having any problems feeding Ami during the night and whether they would like for the dietitian to review the feeding regime. I thought to myself that it must be a difficult task because Ami had a lot of very strong thrashing arm movements and head movements so the tube often came out. Also, I reflected that because both parents were teenagers they might find it difficult to get up during the night for feeds. During another visit we noticed redness on the back of Ami's head and it became apparent that the reason for these was that she was laid on the floor for long periods. Stephanie and Liam took a long time convincing that the redness was caused because her head was thrashing around and rubbing against the hard floor matting. I saw for myself how difficult it was for the nurses to promote a trusting partnership type of relationship with Stephanie and Liam. They had to be so careful how, when and why they gave advice and/or intervened but they also had to be very aware of child protection issues.'

Difficulties for Ami and her family

We thought the following difficulties should be taken into account (you may have come up with more).

+ Ami is a premature baby with complex health needs.
+ Ami has been in hospital for some time and separated from her parents - attachment and bonding will have been affected.
+ There is a possibility of a child at risk.
+ The sparse visiting by Stephanie and Liam may be an indication that they are frightened of having a sick baby and being responsible for her care or may be related to the loss (absence) of a healthy child.
+ Tube feeding has reinforced that the child is sick and different and requires high-level practical skills to care for her.
+ Stephanie has been sleeping rough during the pregnancy, suggesting that she may have very little social support and may still be in need of help to provide a stable, consistent environment.

The challenges for the nurses therefore included:

+ A need for effective risk assessment and to use knowledge about child protection issues and strategies, based on effective multidisciplinary working.
+ Problems in communication with parents in forming a relationship built on trust which is supportive and one in which parenting skills can be taught/learned and monitored.
+ Consideration of what strengths, resources and solutions would be useful.

Caring for Ami therefore involves taking so many aspects into account. We know that some families are resilient and more capable than others in coping with extreme stress and adversity. However, any family faced with the situation of Stephanie and Liam would need help to build up their family strengths and resources. You will find many studies related to family resilience in sociological and psychological literature. Patterson (2002) considers families as a 'social system' built upon a network of interrelationships, values and beliefs. Belonging to a family is a source of physical and psychological nurture and Ami needs to grow up in a family where, amongst other important things, she is loved and kept safe. Communication with Stephanie and Liam, and between all professionals involved in their care, is of vital importance if the family is to be helped to function well. This will include an accurate assessment of their capabilities and of the ways in which they view the situation. Recognising successes, however small, is crucial (Patterson, 2002).

Patterson goes on to call for a 'family strengths approach' to discover assets and resources that will enhance family members' capabilities and ensure that they are not overwhelmed. Stephanie had managed to overcome difficult teenage years and had formed a stable relationship with Liam. This was potentially a good foundation for family life. In addition, Liam's mother proved to be a supportive, well organised and capable family resource to assist with Ami. This focus on strengths, resources and possible solutions rather than only on problems will be discussed again in Chapter 7.

As you can see and may have experienced, helping people like Stephanie and Liam with a very sick child or those who have to adapt to a changed lifestyle following illness or surgery can be very challenging. As well as changes in health behaviour and lifestyle, we may expect service users and carers to master physically complex tasks such as looking after a colostomy, a Hickman catheter, caring for a tracheotomy or learning to live with a urinary catheter. Other families might have to find ways of coping with challenging behaviour, confusion or apathy. Whilst some may be able to adapt or even relish the challenge, for others it might take a great deal of patience on the part of professionals and all our skills in negotiation, teaching, motivation and support to help them succeed. We have to find the right time to introduce new skills and the receptivity of patient or carer will also influence the interactions we have with them (Euswas and Chick, 1999).

Caring and the challenges of concordance

One of the challenges that nurses may face is related to compliance with planned interventions or prescribed medication. Compliance implies that the person has agreed to follow and/ or act in accordance with expectations of what has been suggested, recommended or prescribed. However, if there is not agreement and clear understanding between professional and service users, compliance may not occur. The word 'compliance' itself is problematic and implies unquestioning obedience with no opportunity for choice (Snelgrove, 2006). It is sometimes used interchangeably with 'adherence' but even this suggests a degree of passivity and obedience. Using the word 'concordance' has a less paternalistic connotation. It implies that people should make their own decisions about whether or not to take a prescribed treatment, after hearing about the relative benefits and risks. The benefit of this approach is that if they do so they are then more likely to be committed to taking their medicine or following a treatment plan.

Read the following story concerning a visit by a student nurse and her mentor a few years ago and consider the following:

+ What do you think the nurses would find when they repeated their visit to Connie?

+ What changes in approach might you have tried?

Case Study 5.8

'We were visiting Connie, a 65-year-old lady who is overweight and has a history of chronic venous leg ulcers and cardiovascular disease. She lives with her husband Fred who is in his 70s who looks after her and does most of the cooking and other housework. Connie spends most of her time watching television and doesn't get out much. Her leg ulcers weren't healing so the community nurse asked for help from the tissue viability nurse who visited Connie and advised the community nurse to redress them twice a week and use compression bandaging. Connie was very suspicious about whether this approach would help but both nurses went through the whys and wherefores and eventually she agreed. Two days later when we went in, we found that she'd taken all the bandages off and said that they were 'hot and uncomfortable' and 'making her short of breath'. Fred agreed with her. The community nurse told them that the bandages couldn't be causing the breathlessness and told Connie to persevere. She said that if she kept her legs elevated when she was sitting and tried to walk about a bit more it would help her circulation in general. The bandages were reapplied and we left Connie to try again.'

We expect that, like us, you doubted whether Connie would still have the bandages on her legs when the nurse visited her again. The challenge for nurses is to get Connie to see herself as an equal partner who is sharing in the decision making. For this to occur, a patient and sensitive approach is needed. In an early but significant study, Bland (1999) provides good insights with her investigation into how people experience living with leg ulcers which might help us understand Connie's situation and guide our practice for a more effective outcome. Bland wanted to understand more about the pain and discomfort experienced and how people coped with them. This, as we have seen, is an important aspect of a caring attitude and she needed to get people's stories in order to understand why so many didn't comply with the treatment. She found that some people experienced major problems with wound odour and oozing which sometimes led to lack of compliance with wound management. To cope with the oozing, for example, people padded the wounds even more. Like Connie, some people found that particularly in hot weather the bandaging brought discomfort and was perceived as unsightly, which led to it being removed. The smell also led to feelings of shame and embarrassment and also sometimes affected marriages by leading to a change in sleeping arrangements. People felt ashamed if others had to do the washing, e.g. of bed linen, and were reluctant to stay away from home because of this. There were feelings of being trapped in an imperfect body. Bland (1999) found that pain was often not assessed by the nurses so they were not able to enter into a true partnership with the patient since much of the information they needed to give good and effective care was missing. A caring and holistic approach, considering the psychological and the social impact of the effect of living with a leg ulcer, might have had dramatic effects on the outcome of the care provided. Bland went on to note that 'when the focus of the health professional is on wound management and the focus of the patient is on minimising the impact of what appears to be a permanent condition so he or she can get on with life, compliance can become problematic for the patient' (Bland, 1999:54). Bland stresses the importance of identifying what problems may be in the way of complying with treatments or health-related guidance and in Connie's case an acknowledgement and further exploration of the discomfort she was having might have led to a change in attitude on her part or an agreement about another course of action.

There were similar findings for Bollini *et al.* (2004), who investigated problems of 'adherence' to treatments for people with mental illness and their families. They found some of the problems related to denial of illness, adverse reactions to treatment and lack of clarity about their condition and plans for the future. Forsyth (2007) found another problem concerning the emotional reactions of the nurses and their beliefs about people. He investigated the nature of the nurse–client relationship when an individual has complex problems such as those leading to a diagnosis of a borderline personality disorder (BPD). Engaging with these clients could bring feelings of anger and negativity in the nurse, who judged them as responsible for their own actions and dismissed their behaviour as attention-seeking.

There are parallels for this in other areas of nursing where individuals may be blamed or held responsible for their problems, e.g. those who are overweight, those with smoking- or alcohol-related diseases, or even those, like Connie, with non-healing leg ulcers. Forsyth (2007) stressed the need for reflection on practice so that we articulate and understand our emotions, indicating that this will help us to understand what might be standing in the way of being able to identify the best ways to help clients.

Time to think back

The stories of Ami and Connie have illustrated the challenges of holistic care and creating effective partnerships with carers and those receiving care. They have helped demonstrate that it requires a great deal of patient, skilled observation and ability to identify what problems may lie in the way of working together so that there is concordance in decisions concerning treatments. Ami was at risk because she was vulnerable and her parents needed to develop not only the parenting skills necessary for any child but also those needed for the care of a child with disabilities. Her safety and protection were key areas of concern. This called for a multi-professional and multi-agency approach in order to focus not only on the multiple problems there were but also on the family strengths and resources available, Connie's story also demonstrated why equitable and effective partnerships with service users are essential.

Being out of step

People may feel themselves to be 'out of step' with health professionals and this may give rise to distressing ethical debates. Read Jasmine's story and consider what decision you think staff looking after her may have come to.

Case Study 5.9

Jasmine was 14 years old and had been discharged from hospital. She had been diagnosed at an early age with leukaemia and had been through a number of treatment regimes – the latest had been extensive and had left her and her family feeling negative and emotionally drained. It was apparent that the pressures of living with such an illness were having an increasing effect on Jasmine and her parents. Jasmine also had a two-year-old brother, Thomas, who she enjoyed looking after.

Jasmine made a decision that she no longer wanted to comply with medications and treatments but wanted to live the rest of her life at home with her family. Her parents believed that she had thought things through and made the decision and that there was nothing more they could do in persuading her to comply. Staff in the unit were unhappy and frustrated. They did not want to 'give up the fight' although it seemed that this is what Jasmine and her family wanted.

Although this is a difficult situation, it presents the kind of ethical dilemma you will come across throughout your career, and your academic work related to legal requirements, human rights and ethical theories and frameworks will help you consider these complex practice situations from different standpoints and see how they may be applied to everyday decision making. They also underpin professional standards and the NMC Code of Conduct (2008), which, as a nurse, you are required to follow. To caring professionals, 'letting go' of Jasmine and letting her do as she wishes may seem uncaring, but you may also have thought that not doing so could be considered to be paternalistic, in that staff may be at risk of trying to make decisions on behalf of Jasmine and her family, so not working in concordance with her.

In Jasmine's case, although there were some misgivings initially, medical and nursing staff did not try to challenge the family's decision but shared all the information available to them about the likely consequences of their action so that Jasmine and her family were able to make a well considered and informed choice. Jasmine was able to return home, supported by community staff, and live with her family in the last few months of her life. Jasmine did not want to endure any further treatments. She knew she would die, but made a clear decision that she wanted to do this peacefully at home with her loved ones. Maude and Hawley (2007) remind us that children (as long as they fully understand and are able to make an informed decision) have the same rights as adults. Staff were able to draw on a good relationship, built up over a number of years with both Jasmine and her family, to ensure any decision was well considered. By doing so they may have been guided by the four main principles used to guide ethical practice: autonomy, beneficence, justice and non-maleficence.

In health care, autonomy means that an individual has a right to make their own decisions, e.g. to consent to or refuse treatment. This requires open communication between staff and the patient/client so that they are able to 'deliberate rationally through various possible courses of actions without being impaired by lack of time, incomplete information, mental illness and/or impairment' (Newham and Hawley, 2007:79). Jasmine had time, was informed of the consequences and was able, with her parents, to make a rational decision.

Beneficence means that action is in a patient's best interests – what is seen as beneficial, or good for the well-being of the individual. Providing information and continued support at home helped staff to act in Jasmine's best interest in terms of what she and her family wanted.

Justice is a acting in a way that is fair and equal. Jasmine was given the opportunity to continue a pathway of treatment, as another person in her situation would be, but she chose to refuse it. She was not penalised or discriminated against because of this action but support and help continued.

Non-maleficence refers to 'doing no harm'. It covers not only a duty of care but also the need to avoid both actual harm and the risk of harm (Newham and Hawley, 2007). This could suggest that this principle was not met as without further treatment, her death could be hastened. However, another application of this principle would be to consider that more treatments would cause her suffering, pain and separation from her family.

We hope that this will help you to see that theories and frameworks can be very help-ful. Caring does require critical analysis of difficult situations, particularly those that involve an ethical dilemma and for which we need to reflect on ethical and legal considerations if we are going to be better able to help patients and their families and safeguard ourselves. This is all part of compassionate care. We need all the resources available to help us to do that and acquiring knowledge of principles such as those acquired from ethics will help us a great deal. To be caring means that we should ensure that we are open to new knowledge throughout our professional lives. This is what we mean by lifelong learning.

Some people may also feel isolated or out of step with professionals because of their condition. O'Loughlin (1999) found that people with chronic pain often felt lonely, isolated and fearful and might find themselves labelled as 'the chronic pain patient' with the covert assumption that the pain was 'in the head' and therefore not valid. She described the expe-rience of a patient who had a psychiatric history and felt negative stereotyping occurred because of this. Some health-care professionals, she thought, had the belief that her chronic pain originated from the mind and was therefore illegitimate. As a result she felt dismissed and not valued as a person. She also found there were difficulties for the family. One suf-ferer told her, 'My husband tells me that when you've got chronic pain, you are a chronic pain. He's not trying to be nasty. It's just that that's what it's like to live with someone who has pain all the time' (O'Loughlin, 1999:134).

O'Loughlin found health-care professionals generally had inadequate knowledge of the complexities and effects of living with chronic pain. Pharmacological interventions may be prescribed but she claimed that these might not be the answer if there are side effects which may lead to feelings of frustration and anger, and highlighted the need for a range of measures to assess and treat pain such as the more holistic approach taken within pain clinics. Caring for someone in pain means trying to understand it. Important work by Madjar (1999) indicates that pain relief depends on the experience being shared and so requires visibility – we need language to describe pain. People may try to keep it private and there-fore invisible – they may try to protect others and to keep their composure. The nurse needs to help the patient to describe pain and to share with them in the control of that pain. Madjar (1999) related this to caring, which she defined as paying close attention to human experi-ence but noted that it requires knowledge, skill and sensitivity. A decade on and there is still a need for more skilled responses to the recognition and treatment of pain. An RCN report in 2009 described paediatric pain recognition as inadequate. A contributing factor is children's inability in expressing pain to those taking care of them in a way that is recognised and clearly understood. This is particularly the case if a child or adult has cognitive impairment and highlights the need for nurses to keep up to date with guidance on pain recognition, assessment tools and pain management in whatever branch of nursing they are working. Pain in older people may be dismissed not only by others but by themselves as an inevi-table part of the ageing process. Ageist and discriminatory attitudes towards older people in pain must therefore be challenged, particularly since dignity and pain are interrelated, a view highlighted by the Health Service Commissioner for England (2011). Kumar and Allcock (2008) collected reflections from older people about their experiences of living with pain. Their stories led the authors to conclude that:

'Any effort to deliver dignity in care needs to ensure that no older person suffers pain unnecessarily. To bring this about, the older person must be able to make choices concerning the treatment of their pain and to exert control over how it is managed and who manages it. At the same time, staff should be ensuring that relief of pain is timely and that their own attitudes toward older people are not discriminatory.' (Kumar and Allcock 2008:5)

To think about

+ Can you think of anyone you have cared for who may have thought they were 'out of step' with professionals?
+ What did you do, or might you have done, to help them?
+ Are you up to date with pain assessment and management?

Nurses aren't miracle workers

Sometimes we have to come to terms with the fact that people may have different preoccupations, drives and motives and we may find it very difficult to divert them from what we see as risky or harmful behaviour. Marcus, a community psychiatric nurse, told us of his work with Brett, a 30-year-old man with a 14-year history of substance dependency including injecting heroin into his groin. He also had a complex medical history. He had been treated for deep vein thrombosis, blood-borne infections and was hepatitis C positive. He had little contact with his family and few friends, with his main form of 'support' coming from his drug dealers.

Read the following account of Marcus's intervention with Brett and consider what aspects he might have wanted to reflect upon, both during and after the event.

Case Study 5.10

'I saw my nursing role as one of persuading Brett into treatment to reduce risks mainly around unsafe injecting. This was to be done by substitute prescribing of methadone and key work sessions around harm reduction.

Brett was always difficult to engage. He did not always keep to agreed times of appointments and continued to groin inject. On one occasion, he informed me that he had started taking a solvent. I asked him what this was and he said it was butane gas directly from the can. I was very concerned and told him about the increased risk that he was putting himself in. I tried to explore "triggers" that he felt led him to use the gas and strongly reinforced how dangerous it was. He told me not to worry, that he would be OK. I tried to be realistic in what behaviour he might be expected to change as I knew this was the only way I could get him to listen to me. I suggested that, if he continued to use butane in spite of the risks to himself, it was safer to inhale from a bag rather than directly from the can. I really felt that he had taken this on board. However, this was not the case as he was found dead a week later through inhaling from a can. I felt sad, angry with myself for not being able to prevent it but also very angry with him.'

Compare your considerations with ours

It was obvious to us that Marcus cared greatly about Brett but he had mixed feelings of anger and frustration as well as feelings of sadness. Perhaps he asked himself if he had been caring enough and he would have needed support, which may have come in the form of clinical supervision or debriefing.

Marcus would have considered whether he had used the 'right' approach – and why he was angry and upset. However, it was important for him to reflect that he had drawn on ethical principles to guide his practice, e.g. he tried his best to listen and negotiate with Brett, provided information and a plan of action that he thought might be less risky (even though it was far from an 'ideal' solution). In doing so he was trying to avoid harm coming to Brett as much as he possibly could, given the complex circumstances.

As he failed to influence Brett, Marcus was disappointed with himself (and also with Brett) but we have to come to terms with the fact that we may not always succeed. Reflection can help us with this and we can draw on assistance from literature. According to Narayanasamy (1999), we can facilitate change in others but we should not assume responsibility for that change. Health behaviour is complex. A number of methods can be used to try to help those at risk to change their behaviour, but motivation and the nature and magnitude of the problems the individual faces will play a significant part (Morrison and Bennett, 2006).

Nurses often have very high expectations of themselves although many factors may stand in the way of what they see as 'perfect' practice. Marcus may have what Glasberg *et al.* (2007) describe as the 'troubled conscience' all health-care workers may have when they feel they cannot provide the 'good' care they wish to give.

It is this kind of complex situation that is a problem for nurses 'because as we have seen, professional achievement influences our evaluation of ourselves as caring. Clouder (2005) argues that when student health professionals undergo practice placements, they meet challenges to themselves as caring people and undergo a transformation in their sense of identity. She suggests that caring is a 'threshold concept' because of the 'troublesome knowledge' with which students are confronted. For her, this means that when faced with the reality of practice, students have to revise their thoughts about what they mean by caring since not everyone can be cured or treated, as some interventions may fail; some people may not respond to care or may refuse it. From our experience and as expressed in Marcus's story, it would seem that nurses have to do this in a thoughtful and reflective manner throughout their career, particularly given the number of ethical dilemmas that occur.

Sometimes a situation we encounter helps to keep our feet on the ground. What do you think we can learn from the following?

Case Study 5.11

Peter is a 12-year-old boy who has to have a supra-pubic catheterisation every three to four hours. He has required this since he was a baby because without the catheter he cannot empty his bladder properly and there is a leakage of urine. The nurses in the community have worked with Peter and his family since he was very young. Their input has been varied and very substantial, ranging from catheterising Peter when he was too young to do it himself, to teaching his parents, and then Peter, how to catheterise, liaising with the school to assist with inclusion and confidentiality issues. The school were great and even had a school shower installed for him to discreetly use. None of his school peers knew of this catheterisation issue, so that was never a problem. The school, nursing staff and parents were all so supportive towards Peter and worked very well together to get everything sorted for him. When he was about 10 or 11 years old, Peter declared he was not bothered whether he was wet or dry. He would not catheterise himself and chose to wear an incontinence pad. Everyone tried to get Peter to change his mind. For example, at school he was reminded about the catheterisation when due, and of course the staff members were very discreet so that his peers did not know. The nurses did body image and self-esteem work and so on. This was to no avail and went on for well over a year. The multidisciplinary team's anxiety was very high and the staff and Peter's parents were in despair, saying they just did not know what to do next. Eventually, Peter's psychologist told them that it was their problem and not Peter's and that until Peter wanted to conform there was little left to do. This did not seem to help anyone's anxiety or frustration!

Earlier this week Peter's mother phoned the nursing team, both laughing and crying. She said, 'You will never believe this and I feel awful about what I said to Peter but it seems to have worked. Peter is now suddenly self-catheterising and is very proud of being clean and dry. I was so desperate and angry so I said to him, "Girls don't like dirty little boys like you."' That stopped him in his tracks and he has certainly changed his behaviour now. All of your hard work and that is what did the trick!

This story reiterates the points made earlier about the importance of timing and receptivity of the patient. Peter had reached a stage in his life where his appearance and the way he was perceived by others (especially girls) mattered to him. His mother, exasperated and frustrated, inadvertently pressed the 'right' button! The last two stories have illustrated that we need to be realistic about what we can achieve and when. There may not be immediate answers or solutions. Working together with patients and their families requires patience and working towards maintenance of trust within professional boundaries.

Summary

In this chapter we have seen the importance and necessity of creating effective partnerships with carers and those receiving care. Holistic, compassionate care is not easy within changing political, economic and social contexts but can be helped if we work closely with relatives and their families in identifying not only problems but also family strengths and resources. Recognition that, as professionals, we are often only one small part of a continuum of care will make us more alert to the importance of ensuring that we work with informal carers. We have seen the importance of continuity of care. Patient and carer participation in care evaluations, forums and services such as PALS (**www.pals.nhs.uk**) all help to do this, but in everyday practice we must make sure we enter into effective dialogue with service users and their carers. Paying attention to what people say about their lived experiences of illness or disability, of providing care and being cared for, will help us to bring into effect the most important aspect of nursing, that of truly caring partnerships.

Looking forward

To develop our capacity to be caring in our care, and demonstrate compassion, we need to learn more about others and also about ourselves. In the next chapter we will focus on how we might further develop ourselves and our therapeutic relationships.

Activity

One of the care indicators you will see at the end of this chapter refers to looking for and knowing about resources.

+ How do you keep up to date with all the changing government policies?
+ Do you help service users and carers to do this?

Caring indicators

1. Forming relationships with individuals and their families based on trust
2. Helping individuals build up a sense of personal and social worth, acceptability and hope, in order to foster resilience and capability
3. Respecting the privacy of the family and their right to make decisions about and participate in the care, establishing equitable and non-patronising partnerships
4. Helping carers to avoid 'care overload' by assisting them to change distressing situations into manageable ones
5. Being alert to client 'readiness' by recognising the time to give supportive help and information, including those with cognitive impairment
6. Not making assumptions but listening to what people say, including children, paying attention to how they describe their situation and their lived experience
7. Understanding the needs of individuals and their carers by using skills of negotiation, motivation, teaching and support to help them succeed
8. Engaging in effective risk assessment, using legal, ethical and academic knowledge to help safeguard patients, families and ourselves
9. Engaging in effective multi-professional, multi-agency care, making patient and carers of central importance
10. Coordinating successful transitions between health and social care sectors, recognising as professionals we are part of a continuum of care

Further reading

The Department of Health website on **www.dh.gov.uk**. In its publications section you will be able to keep up to date with government policies and guidelines and also information which will be useful for carers, such as the booklet entitled *Information and Support for the Carers of People with Dementia.*

You can download a toolkit and supplementary resources which highlight good practice in involving people with dementia in service planning, delivery and evaluation. This has been developed by the National Mental Health Development Unit with the help of patients and their carers and can be found at **www.nhmdu.org.uk** (last accessed 14/03/2012). Insert 'strengthening involvement' into the search engine.

The Public Service website: **www.direct.gov.uk**
The Carers' website: **www.carersuk.org**
The Dementia Support Group website: **www.dementialink.org**
The Social Care Institute for Excellence website on **www.scie.org.uk** has quick and easy access to key research and policies and also ideas from practice.

References

Aggarwal, N, Vass, A, Minardi, H, Ward, R, Garfield, C and Cybyk, B (2003) People with dementia and their relatives: personal experiences of Alzheimer's and of the provision of care. *Journal of Psychiatric and Mental Health Nursing* **10**, 187-197.

Aldridge, J and Becker, S (2003) *Children Caring for Parents with Mental Illness: Perspectives of young carers, parents and professionals.* London: The Policy Press.

BBC (2010) *Cameron wars on child carer cuts.* Available at **bbc.co.uk/news/education-11757907** (last accessed on 13/03/2010).

Bland, M (1999) *On living with leg ulcers.* In Madjar, I and Walton, J (eds) *Nursing and the Experience of Illness: Phenomenology in practice.* London and New York: Routledge.

Bollini, P, Tibaldi, G, Testa, C and Munizza, C (2004) Understanding treatment adherence in affective disorders: a qualitative study. *Journal of Psychiatric and Mental Health Nursing* **11**,668-674.

Brouwer, W, Van Excel, N, Van den Berg, B, Van den Bos, G and Koopmanschap, M (2005) Process utility from providing informal care: the benefit of caring. *Health Policy* **74**, 85-99.

Clouder, L (2005) Caring as a 'threshold concept' transforming students in higher education into health (care) professionals. *Teaching in Higher Education* **10**, 505-517.

DOH (Department of Health) (2008) *Carers at the heart of 21st Century families and communities.* Available at: **dh.gov.uk/publications**. (last accessed 06/03/2012).

DOH (Department of Health (2009) *Report of the Standing Commission on Carers 2007 to 2009.* Available online at: **dh.gov.uk/publications**. (last accessed 16/04/2012).

DOH (Department of Health) (2010) *Recognized, valued and supported. Next steps for the National Carers Strategy.* Available at: **dh.gov.uk/publication**. (last accessed 06/03/2012).

Euswas, P and Chick, N (1999) On caring and being cared for. In Madjar, I and Walton, J (eds) *Nursing and the Experience of Illness: Phenomenology in Practice.* London and New York: Routledge.

Forsyth, A (2007) The effects of diagnosis and non-compliance attributions on therapeutic alliance processes in adult acute psychiatric settings. *Journal of Psychiatric and Mental Health Nursing* **14**, 33-40.

Francis, R (2010) *Independent Inquiry into care provided by Mid-Staffordshire NHS Foundation Trust January 2005 – March 2009*. London: Stationery Office.

Glasberg, A, Erikson, S and Norberg, A (2007) Burnout and 'stress of conscience' among health care personnel. *Journal of Advanced Nursing* **57**, 392–403.

Health Service Commissioner for England (2011) Report of the Health Ombudsman on 10 investigations into NHS care of older people. London: Stationery Office.

Kitwood, T (1997) *Dementia Reconsidered – the Person comes First*. Buckingham: Open University Press.

Kumar, A and Allcock, N (2008) *Pain in older people. Reflections and experiences from an older person's perspective*. Available at: **www.britishpainsociety.org/book_pain_in_older_age_ID7826.pdf** (last accessed 16/04/2012).

Madjar, M (1999) *On inflicting and relieving pain*. In Madjar, I and Walton, J (eds) *Nursing and the Experience of Illness: Phenomenology in Practice*. London and New York: Routledge.

Maude, P and Hawley, G (2007) *Clients' and patients' rights and protecting the vulnerable*. In Hawley, G (ed) *Ethics in Clinical Practice*. Harlow: Pearson Education.

Morrison, V and Bennett, P (2006) *An Introduction to Health Psychology*. Harlow: Pearson Education.

Narayanasamy, A (1999) Learning spiritual dimensions of care from a historical perspective. *Nurse Education Today* **19**, 386–39.

Newham, N and Hawley, G (2007) The relationship of ethics to philosophy. In Hawley, G (ed) *Ethics in Clinical Practice*. Harlow: Pearson Education.

NMC (Nursing and Midwifery Council) (2008) *The Code: Standards of conduct, performance and ethics for nurses and midwives*. London: Nursing and Midwifery Council.

O'Loughlin, A (1999) On living with chronic pain. In Madjar, I and Walton, J (eds) *Nursing and the Experience of Illness: Phenomenology in practice*. London and New York: Routledge.

Patterson, J (2002) Understanding family resilience. *Journal of Clinical Psychology* **58**, 233–246.

Phillips, J, Bernard, M and Chittenden, M (2002) *Juggling Work and Care: The experiences of working carers of older adults*. London: The Policy Press.

Princess Royal Trust for Carers and Crossroads for Caring (2009) *Putting People First without Putting Carers Second* Available at: **www.carers.org/professionals/health/health-and-wellbeing,808,PP.html** (last accessed 11/03/2012).

Skills for Care, Skills for Health, Department of Health (2011) *Common core principles for supporting people with dementia: a guide to training the social care and health workforce* Available at: **www.dhgov.uk/publications** (last accessed 06/03/2012).

Snelgrove, S (2006) Factors contributing to poor concordance in health care. *Nursing Times,102,2,28*. Available at: **nursing times.net**. (last accessed 13/03/2012).

Spencer, J, Godolphin, W, Karpenko, N, Towle, A (2011) *Can patients be teachers? Involving patients and service users in healthcare professionals' education*. The Health Foundation. Available at: **www. health.org.uk** (last accessed 22/01/ 2012).

Witton, M (2003) Support act. *Nursing Standard* **18**, 14–15.

Witucki-Brown, J, Chen, S, Mitchell, C and Province, A (2007) Help-seeking by older husbands caring for wives with dementia. *Journal of Advanced Nursing* **59**, 352–360.

Yeandle, S, Bennett, C, Buckner, L, Fry, G, Price, C (2007) *Stages and Transitions in the Experience of Caring*. Carers UK. Available at: **www.carersuk.org**. (last accessed 16/04/2012).

Chapter 6
Transformative learning – being and becoming

LEARNING OBJECTIVES

By the end of this chapter you should have an understanding of how:

1. Accessing and analysing our emotions can help us to learn more about ourselves and influence our therapeutic relationships

2. Self-awareness and self-regard can influence our interactions with others and our potential to learn

3. Reflective strategies including the use of metaphors can increase our understanding of self and others

4. Role modelling and sharing expertise help with the development of caring skills

5. Support networks such as clinical supervision, mentorship and preceptorship are important for enhancing our caring skills and influencing our personal and professional development

Introduction

In this chapter we shall consider how we can learn more about ourselves by understanding our emotions and how we might use them to develop our capacity to be caring in our care. We will use examples from practice to discuss how reflection can increase our self-awareness and consider the ways in which we might be analytical about ourselves using metaphors and images to help us understand ourselves more. We will also explore the notion of emotional intelligence and its place in our professional development. We will discuss the impact of changes in health care on therapeutic nurse–patient relationships and what we can do to maintain and enhance caring approaches through sharing our skills and expertise.

What our emotions do for us

In previous chapters we have discussed how it may sometimes seem as if our emotions are more of a hindrance than a help. They can cloud our judgement and our performance. We can be accused of being too emotional at times, in our everyday relationships as well as at work. It may mean we become too attached and upset by situations, react unthinkingly to what people say or do, or forget what we are supposed to be doing as we are so preoccupied with our own feelings. If we are to be caring, it is important to consider what our emotions tell us about ourselves and how we can best access them and learn from them. In nursing, increasing our self-awareness is seen as an important requisite for therapeutic interactions and critical reflection, but first of all it seems appropriate to think about what we mean by the self. Understanding ourselves is not an easy task as we are all complex individuals.

Stevens (1996) suggests there are five aspects that help us understand what it means to be a person. It involves physical embodiment – we have a body with physiological sensations and responses, which, as we know, may be prone to disease, stress and pain and which affect the way we perceive ourselves and are perceived by others. It also involves subjective experience as we use our ability to initiate thoughts and actions and make sense of our experience through our cognitive or thought processes. However, a third aspect is that we live in a social world so we are 'linked to others and exist in a social medium of meanings and customs' (Stevens, 1996:16). This is a strong influence on our values, beliefs and prejudices, as we are influenced by what we think is expected in our behaviour and attitudes (social norms). We know this is important in nursing, not only because of how we are socialised into it and perceive ourselves as nurses, but also because we are aware of the influence of cultural and religious beliefs on how patients feel about themselves and the ways in which they experience illness. Another set of influences on our self-perceptions is the likelihood of unconscious or hidden thoughts and feelings that may occur as a result of previous experiences. Those adopting a psychodynamic approach, for example, emphasise the mechanisms we use to defend our ego (or sense of self) such as repression, denial and projection, which we use in everyday life and may all act as barriers to self-knowledge. Lastly, Stevens highlights the important effect on us of the inter-relationship of all of the above. In other words, he identifies the impact of a complex range of influencing factors on the way we perceive ourselves. This calls for a great deal of 'intelligence' so we are able to detect the influences of our own predispositions, characteristics, values and prejudices in our relationships with others if we are to be able to understand them and interact effectively with them. As you will see later in this chapter we will draw on an approach in which each individual is seen as an agent (in other words a manager) of their own social construction – this involves an active and changing process (Wetherall and Maybin, 1996).

A sense of personal identity, body image, role performance and self-esteem are all aspects of self-awareness (Kozier et al., 2008) and influence whether or not we have a positive view of ourselves. Our identity is a combination of physical and personality characteristics, values, beliefs and perceptions of our body image and our capabilities. These are all linked to how we regard ourselves in terms of self-esteem and role performance (e.g. as a mother, brother, friend, practitioner). Our self-concept changes as a result of development, our experiences, illness and stress. We have an image of ourselves as an 'ideal' person but all too often we fall short of this.

Students and newly qualified nurses go through particular challenging periods of learning and change. During these times it is easy to focus on aspects you feel negative about, but you also need to consider your strengths and how you can develop them further. This is because a positive self-concept is essential to our mental and physical health. It helps us to adapt and cope with change: in other words, to be more resilient. If we are positive about ourselves, we are also more likely to be able to help others (as long as we are honest and do not go to the other extreme of always excusing ourselves and only seeing ourselves in a favourable light). However, being self-aware and honest with ourselves is not easy. It requires courage, confidence, a certain degree of maturity and the support of others (Atkins, 2004). If we develop skills in self-analysis we will be able to evaluate our interactions, responses, behaviours and skills without feeling hopeless or worthless. This means applying the skills of critical analysis to ourselves – looking for a balanced judgement – highlighting the good points as well as the aspects we might need to develop or change. Thompson (2003: 133) emphasises that this process 'is not about self-indulgence or the emotional equivalent to navel-gazing but rather a more positive and constructive emphasis on self-awareness'.

We can develop self-awareness in a variety of ways but doing so takes time and energy. According to Thompson (2003) we can do this by adopting a more conscious and reflective approach as we go about our interactions with others and also by observing interactions between others. He suggests that the more we observe, concentrate and listen attentively, the more aware we can become and the more we can learn. We know that people with sensory deficits, hearing or visual difficulties, can develop extraordinary perceptual abilities in their other senses. There is therefore potential in all of us to develop our sensory capabilities. This will increase our ability to pick up cues or grasp the meaning in encounters with others, which is 'based on a capacity that involves the external senses as well as imagination' – an essential component of the art of nursing (Johnson, 1996:251).

There are exercises designed to help us develop both physical and emotional self-awareness that may be undertaken as an individual, with a partner or as a member of a group (e.g. Thompson, 2002; Atkins, 2004). However, our everyday thinking or introspection also plays a large part in the way in which our self-image and self-knowledge evolve. If we go through a particularly emotional experience in practice we may go over and over in our minds how we, or others, behaved and relive the feelings involved. Memories such as these can last for a very long time. Reflecting on our experiences can help us to analyse and change our perceptions. Some people find that keeping a personal reflective journal or diary is useful for this as it helps to externalise, articulate and review these feelings. Reflection therefore becomes the challenging aspect of memory. It makes us look again at what we have experienced and think about how we reacted. It helps to consider whether our input to a situation was effective by congratulating ourselves on what we think we did well but also noticing what gaps there might be in our knowledge or skills. This can provide us with the incentive to take any appropriate action needed for improvement and to consider what resources we might use to do this. This is why reflection has become so important in nursing. Duke (2004) has provided clear evidence of how reflection can become a vital and integral part of our ongoing professional lives, outlining how it helped her to establish and develop her new role as a nurse consultant.

As we have said, there is a tendency for us, particularly when in a new situation, to focus on our limitations. There is a continual dialogue going on within us as we talk to ourselves about what is going on, what we make of it and how we should respond. Sometimes there may be feelings of panic as we try to find the best thing to say or do. There is an indication of the complexity of this inner speech in the following story written by Sophie, a student nurse undertaking her first practice placement (Smith, 2003). Read her story and think about the following

+ What phrases in the story are significant to help us understand her feelings?

+ What did she learn about herself?

Case Study 6.1

'We pulled up in her car outside a house close to the sea. The community nurse told me we were visiting a lady in her early thirties, married with young children. She had breast cancer, had had treatment but secondaries had occurred in several parts of her body. She was terminally ill and receiving palliative care from the community nurse. A Macmillan nurse was also in attendance. Upon knocking at the door, I wondered what I might expect her to look and act like. Her sister opened the door, greeted us and directed us to the bedroom. Entering the bedroom, I noticed that the patient looked very depressed but she gave us a quick smile. My mentor engaged her in conversation. She answered with brief "yes" or "no" answers.

After 10 minutes of myself casually smiling, occasionally, my mentor informed me she was going back to the car. She had forgotten an enema. A sudden dread came over me! I was going to be left alone with this lady who I didn't know at all. What was I going to say? I quickly tried to think of something to say. The silence seemed awful. Maybe I should mention the weather. Oh no! That's silly – everyone talks about the weather. How boring! What did the weather matter to her, she wasn't going out anywhere, she was so ill. Then I thought about asking her about Christmas, perhaps asking if her family were all prepared. Oh no, I thought – that's worse – she won't be expected to live that long. That might depress her even more.

My mind went blank. I felt awful panicking inside. I quickly gazed round the room, then out of the window, groping for some inspiration. Then I finally saw it – the beautiful sea from her window. That seemed a safe thing to say, I thought. I commented on the lovely view and how it reminded me of a house I used to live in, in Berwick-upon-Tweed, facing the sea. She smiled and said it was lovely. At that moment my mentor came back into the room and I sighed with relief. The nurse resumed her conversation and I never spoke again until it was time to say goodbye.'

Compare your considerations with ours

We can learn a great deal by looking at Sophie's story closely and the language she used. She disclosed a great deal about herself – her thoughts and feelings. Her apprehension is reflected in her initial questioning about what a terminally ill patient might 'look and act like'. The story then goes on to provide a vivid insight into the way in which she searched for the 'right words' to say, and helps to understand the turmoil the student felt after being left on her own. You may have experienced this. Her use of phrases such as 'a sudden dread came over me', 'that would be silly' and the active 'groping for some inspiration', illustrate both her feelings of insecurity and the internal turmoil of her thoughts and feelings. She felt extremely vulnerable and she had to work hard to find the right words to say and yet appear calm. This is an example of emotional labour as described in previous chapters.

Initially, Sophie was conscious of the need to feel part of the exchange between her mentor and the patient by 'casually smiling' but the responsibility shifted significantly when she was left alone. She was aware of the silence, which she felt she must break and her consideration and consequent dismissal of what she saw as inappropriate topic areas added to her anxiety. She was also pleased that eventually she managed to find an answer and her relief was evident.

You may have found that, like us, you think that Sophie told the story to demonstrate the difficulties associated with being left alone and therefore responsible for communicating effectively with a terminally ill patient, an area of experience new to her. We followed her pathway of thinking and feelings as she told us details of her attempts to be caring and how she tried to avoid causing distress. She also indicated her relief when she found a solution to her problem. Overall, in spite of her misgivings, she seemed pleased that she managed to find the 'right' words to say.

There are many ways in which Sophie's reflection on this experience would have helped increase her self-awareness and better understand what she could and did learn from it. Writing her story down, just as she recalled it, capturing her thoughts and feelings, provided a focus for further exploration. She could then have used a reflective model to guide her thoughts even further and analyse her behaviour. A variety of frameworks may be used to guide this, e.g. Gibbs's reflective cycle (Gibbs, 1988) or Johns's more structured approach (Johns, 2000).

In fact, the story was used as a focus for peer group discussion in which the student received positive support for the way in which she coped with the situation. It also provided an important opportunity for a group discussion about perceptions of what was 'appropriate' subject matter in conversing with dying patients, including the use of silence in communication. Further exploration of the literature about these areas helped all the students clarify and extend their learning by integrating practice and theory. The theory helped illuminate their practice.

To think about

+ Write about a situation when you felt at a loss because you didn't know what to say or do (we all have them!). Write it as if you were writing a letter or an email to a close friend or an entry in your diary.
+ Look again at the language you use and underline phrases or words that show the emotions you felt. Then consider what you can learn from these about yourself and the way you respond in difficult situations.
+ You can deepen your analysis by linking issues that you discover with academic literature or theories, e.g. related to communication or the use of silence in interactions. This way you can see how what you have learned from your emotional responses has increased your understanding of issues arising in practice and has benefits for the way you manage your feelings and actions in the future.

We hope that the exercise helped you to describe, identify and analyse some of the thoughts and feelings that may occur as we undertake emotional work (or labour) within everyday practice. Becoming more self-aware has been described as the fundamental aspect of emotional intelligence (EI), which is the ability to recognise and use emotional information (Goleman, 1995; Orbach, 1999; Riggio and Reichard, 2008). McQueen (2004:102) identifies the relevance of this to nursing, highlighting an important relationship between emotional intelligence and emotional labour, adding that 'the interpretation of emotional expression and intelligent response in the application of appropriate professional skills, such as emotional work, empathy and counselling skills, can result in patients' emotional states being modified and anxiety ameliorated'. We have seen how this can occur in many of the case studies within this text – for example, in the story of Harry and Rashida (in Chapter 1).

The emotional part of learning

There is an emotional aspect to our learning that may not make sense immediately but sometime after. In Chapter 4, we considered how our reactions to situations can be triggered by significant objects or events that make us think again about what we are seeing. The 'penny drops' and what we have experienced makes more sense. Consider this story about a visit to Frank by a student and her mentor and think about what we can learn from it.

Case Study 6.2

'On this particular day, I was out with the community nurse and we were visiting Frank, who had a long history of alcohol abuse and self-neglect. The nurse warned me to expect some bad language and poor living conditions before we got there. It wasn't as bad as I expected. When we arrived we found Frank sitting in a hole-riddled settee with springs poking through, wearing either his only or favourite suit by the look of it. The floor was quite littered with empty bottles and scrunched-up cans. Frank was suffering from some kind of skin condition (I cannot remember what) due to his appalling diet or should I say lack of it. We treated his legs and got up to go. As we were leaving, the nurse asked him if he would have a shave before her next visit. I remember wondering why she had done this as I know there was no way he could actually get around to doing it. I didn't ask because I thought it would probably seem trivial to the nurse, but I always wanted to ask her if he did have that shave.

It wasn't until some months later that I thought about this again. I was doing some directed reading for once, on self-care. There was a question in the chapter asking you to think of an incident where there was a client with a lifestyle that was concerning and what the philosophy of care was when approaching this subject. Suddenly this memory sprung to mind and I realised what my mentor had been trying to achieve and how it related to what I had been reading. By *asking* this man to have a shave, not only was she encouraging him to take an interest in his lifestyle, she was giving him an option. This was much more ethical than just hanging in there and making him shave, either himself or doing it for him. No matter how good your intentions are for someone, this would surely undermine them and make them feel powerless and useless like a child. By giving this man an option he would not only feel better himself for taking an interest in his hygiene, but he would feel empowered as he was in control of how much care he received and who administered it. OK, this short-term boost probably wouldn't put him on the road back to recovery and make his life worth living again but it would show him that he is always capable of making things a little bit better . . . step by step . . . if only he chose to do so . . . '

Compare your considerations with ours

The story reminds us of the importance of the detail of description because it helps to begin the process of critical reflection. It can help if we look again at the student's story and try to précis it. She describes how a learning situation begins when she is reminded how a patient's condition and appearance are related to his lifestyle, although the situation does not seem as bad as she might have imagined. She questions why her mentor requested something that she thought was unlikely to happen (the shave), but does not ask for an explanation at the time since she thinks the nurse would probably think it was trivial. She recalls her question some time after by reading about self-care and realises what the nurse was trying to achieve by seeing a relationship between her experience and the literature. She is then able to attach value to the approach used by her mentor.

We can again look at the language she was using to get clues about what she was feeling. 'It wasn't until some months later' conveys the importance to her of the time gap between the incident and the reflection. The words 'suddenly this memory sprung to mind' provide an indication of the abrupt clarity with which she is then able to see the situation. She emphasises the word 'asking' to underline her understanding of why the nurse gave Frank a choice. She seems pleased at being able to make the connection with theory and therefore able to explain to herself what happened, but the ending suggests her fear that effecting any change in the patient's lifestyle is likely to be a hard struggle.

Once more, this story provides an important message about how we learn about ourselves and the part reflection might play in that. It is an ongoing process as we try to learn from our experiences and link practice and theory. In this case the theory helped the student to understand an experience. Learning can be described as fitting the pieces of the jigsaw together. Sometimes it isn't until certain pieces are fitted together that we understand what the whole picture is about.

Learning from the language of metaphors

We used the metaphor of the jigsaw to help convey what we thought learning was all about. By encapsulating an image of feelings about an event, that image helps us to see things in a new light; in other words, it helps to uncover hidden aspects. Like similes and images, metaphors are perhaps often thought of as a feature of literature, but are in reality very much part of our everyday lives. The student in the story of Frank, for example talks about words 'springing to mind'. You may remember that a simile occurs when we use the word 'like' or 'as', such as when we ask, 'Does my skin look like a dried-up prune from too much sun?' We use metaphors as a figure of speech when we compare things, highlighting similarities, usually by saying one thing is another, e.g. 'She is a tower of strength.' An example of this is Rebecca's description of how she felt during a 'nurse handover' that took place at the foot of her bed on the first morning after her hip replacement. 'Without looking at me, the night nurse informed the rest of the staff gathered round my bed that I had had a good night. I felt like a "cardboard cut-out" and said very loudly, "Excuse me, I have *not had a good night.*" The metaphor she used summarised very vividly how she was feeling.

Throughout the ages and across civilisations, symbols, images and metaphors have been used in many ways as a form of communication about everyday life, as well as employed in a variety of spiritual, healing and religious practices. They are often a shorthand way of saying something and can help us make sense of our world by projecting rich and complex information that can appeal to a number of our senses – sight, hearing, smell and so on. Education, health care and social work, business and organisational management are some of the communities that, in many different ways, recognise the power of similes, images and metaphors (Graham, 1995). They speak directly to our 'emotional mind'. For example, an advertiser may use a particular image as a way of engaging our unconscious associations – the picture of a person in a white coat holding a specific product might suggest, albeit at a subconscious level, that the product has scientific value and associations.

Sontag (1991) illustrates how military metaphors have, for a long time, been used in medicine as ways of expressing the processes and outcomes of disease – terms such as 'invasion of the body', 'war against disease' and 'victory over cancer' are some such metaphors. It is interesting, however, that Sontag (1991:180) also warns about the use of metaphor in that it can 'powerfully contribute to the excommunicating and stigmatising of the ill'. She illustrates this by referring to a time when the AIDS virus was called the 'gay plague' and it was evident that the metaphor took on moralistic overtones. You may have heard patients describing the phlebotomist as 'Dracula' and Madjar and Walton (1999:9) use a vivid description of staff 'harpooning' for blood when taking arterial gases and link this to a deeply felt experience that pictures both the weapon used and the action taken.

Watson (1999), discusses their use within the context of nursing. 'It is important that the metaphors we employ or accept are made explicit so that we may better understand how they affect our seeing and being. They can be helpful or destructive. They can be unexpected or subtle parallels or analogies. They can encapsulate and put forward proposals or another way of looking at our reality or a given phenomenon' (page 12). Therefore by noticing the metaphors both we and patients use, we can increase our understanding. Many people who have suffered from mental illness have tried to describe their experiences to others in terms of what others might find familiar. Roger, who suffered from periods of depression, was trying to tell his son what depression was like to help him understand. He said he felt like 'a deflated football – all the bounce has gone'. These images are very powerful and help our understanding and therefore increase our empathy. They can also give an insight into our own perceptions, e.g. of growing older. In a collection of poems and writing, written at a creative writing session by older people and staff from a variety of services, getting older in our society was described as being separated from the rest of the community. They described older people as like house plants that are only cared about when they need watering and then instead of being given a good long drink out comes the plant spray and all they get is the first watering of consideration.

As well as helping ourselves to gain more understanding, metaphors can also be a useful way of helping others, for example someone who is struggling to cope with extreme grief. Talking on a radio programme, a father described how, after the suicide of his son, he was helped by a priest who told him that it would seem as if he was always carrying a burden on his back but that, with experience, he would find different ways of carrying that burden. The use of the metaphor helped him see that the priest understood that he would never 'get over' his grief but gave him hope in being able to cope with it in the future.

The following story drawn from our own experience will, we hope, help you understand a little more about the potential for the use of metaphors in understanding, influencing and transforming practice. The case that follows was taken from a clinical supervision session, which was used as a support strategy based on the premise that, in order to care for patients, nurses need to feel cared for themselves.

Case Study 6.3

'Our role was to help support the nurses on the nursing development unit (NDU) and the staff who wished to review their work to date and their professional role to determine what they thought was working well and where they wanted to 'go next' in their developmental process. We were acting as facilitators and knew that a number of authors suggest that the use of metaphors can help us think imaginatively about people and organisations, so we asked the staff if they would consider this. Although they thought this 'a bit academic' they agreed to try it out.

It was interesting, because metaphors (you have to listen for them) were used a great deal during our meetings. Some of the staff said that working in the nursing development unit was stressful because everyone seemed to be watching them; it was like "working in a goldfish bowl" – because of the research funding the unit was receiving. The nurses were very conscious that "the paperwork was very demanding". They said they found it stressful because they believed totally in patient-centred, holistic care and a major theme of their discussions was that they really wanted to focus completely on "hands-on care to do their very best for each patient". It was difficult to get all of the paperwork done as this detracted from their caring role. "Paperwork is important: we need to protect ourselves and cover our backs."

The issue that came up time and time again was about the "nursing boundaries", or, rather, lack of them. To give an example: at one of the meetings the discussion was led by a nurse who introduced the notion of "difficult" patients and relatives. This nurse used the words: "They are difficult, you know those people who want you to dance to their tune." For example, one patient "refused to sleep at night, preferring to position themselves at the nursing desk and talk non-stop for ten hours to the night staff and then sleep during the day". Another nurse told of how a relative of an ill patient had continuously followed her to the canteen and talked to her about the patient all through her lunch and tea breaks. Staff said that they thought the hospital trust had not realised that nurses needed to get away from relatives when it allowed members of the public access to the canteen as a means of income generation. Someone noted that there are ways of avoiding these "difficult" patients and relatives in the canteen and pointed to one of the group members, saying, "You do it by walking fast and looking at the floor."

As facilitators of the session, we highlighted the keywords they were using – the metaphor " . . . those people who want you to dance to their tune". We then used extended metaphors as a way of helping the group examine various alternative scenarios in order for the nurses to feel supported but in which relationships could be more therapeutic:

"What would it be like if patients/relatives were to dance to your tune?"

"What would it be like for the patients/relatives to dance to their own tune and you ignored them?"

"What would it be like for nurses and patients/relatives to dance to their own tunes at the same time?"

"And if the tunes were totally different for nurse/patient/relative?"

This was followed by the question:

"Would it be possible to agree to a tune to which both nurse and patient/relative could dance: to make a joint melody?"'

It was by using these extended metaphors that these nurses came to acknowledge that they needed to learn how to cope with boundaries. There was recognition that all nurses sometimes have a misunderstanding that one's own self-needs must always be subordinated to the needs of others. Emotional and physical labour and issues related with 'burn-out' (feeling physically and emotionally exhausted) were noted.

From this perspective they went on to explore ways of negotiating 'boundaries and limitations' that enabled a trusting, caring relationship characterised by power sharing, empathy and mutuality in the contracting of boundaries. A variety of theoretical perspectives were introduced to the practitioners for them to further consider potential new ways of working. These included Berne's work on transaction analysis (Berne, 1968), which is about analysing and working with various communication styles – such as the nurturing and critical parent, adult and child transactions. Assertion skills and adult-to-adult styles of communication were discussed. The metaphors also provided direction for their reflections and opened up different possibilities for practice. Engaging in this reflective process seemed to help the nurses on the NDU gain a better understanding of some of their options for different ways of working. In other words, it had the potential to help them to be emancipated (more open and less constrained in their thinking) and was likely to transform their ways of thinking and behaving in the future.

To think about

+ Think of metaphors that might describe the nature of a particular aspect of nursing practice. Time is an important element. Try to think of metaphors you could use that might describe your experience of this within practice.
+ Think of the metaphors a patient or client might use about this.

Compare your responses with those found in a research study. Smith (2003) described the metaphors students used. The most common metaphors and vivid descriptions related to time including notions of time flying or time standing still. Time was seen by both students and qualified nurses in their first two years following graduation as a valuable resource but also as a hard taskmaster. There were problems if time was wasted, if they were not given enough time to perform a task or if they took too long over one (as experienced by the graduate who compared unfavourably the length of time she took to give out medicines with her colleagues). There were descriptions of altered experience of time with 'time standing still' or 'dragging' and a minute 'seeming like an eternity' as when students tried to think of what to say 'to fill the silence' or a newly qualified nurse waited for a more senior colleague to relieve her from an onerous responsibility. Time was a commodity that had to be managed and could be given (to patients) or taken (as 'time out' or 'five minutes for yourself'), providing an important way of coping with the job. There were 'not enough hours in the day' to do all they wanted to do, so participants felt guilty as they wanted to 'spend time' with someone and there was 'no time' available. As the students became more senior and following graduation the references to time increased. There were notions of 'running behind' and struggles to 'keep up' with everything. If the pace increased, participants could be 'flying around', 'running around in circles' or 'chasing your tail all day'.

You may have considered that sometimes, cut off from the normal flow of everyday life, time could move slowly for patients. Students in Smith's study described how patients had 'time on their hands' to worry and often had to play 'the waiting game'. One patient who had to deal with an unpredictable and life-threatening condition was described as a 'walking time bomb'. By thinking about the experience of patients in this way, we are able to 'connect' with their experiences in an empathetic way. This will help us to be more caring in our approaches. It can also help us to be more empathetic with ourselves and our colleagues.

You may think, for example, that you are the only one to be experiencing certain neg-ative feelings but you may find parallels in the metaphors students in Smith's study used about their experiences of nursing practice. They sometimes 'felt on the outside' or even a 'nobody', as 'spare parts' or 'intruders' or 'easy targets'. They were worried about being 'thrown in at the deep end' or being 'out of their depth'. As they went through the pro-gramme, there was a requirement to do 'a balancing act' to cope with the 'tension of being a professional and remaining a person'. In the early stages following registration, most felt the stress of 'trying to find one's feet', 'being on the ball', being 'first in the firing line' and 'fit-ting in', but when help came or responsibility was taken on by someone else it felt as if 'a ton was lifted'. When they became the 'blue dress' and the 'buck stopped' they felt they should be able to cope with 'anything thrown your way'. In spite of the undoubted stress and 'prob-lems taken home' there were also positive images of 'enjoying the buzz' and 'thriving on the new-found accountability'.

Metaphors also helped identify other emotional experiences of nursing as participants encountered situations that made them 'fume' or feel 'emotionally drained'. They were wor-ried about 'going over the top', 'flying off the handle' or suffering from 'burn-out'. They needed to stand back from situations and 'switch off' or 'become detached'. They were liable to go into 'overdrive' with 'the adrenaline rushes', 'live on the adrenaline' or, conversely, go onto 'automatic pilot'. There were images relating to extreme emotions such as 'tearing your hair out' or having your 'worst nightmares come true', signifying that they had to find a way of 'letting off steam' or 'sounding off' or they might 'bottle things up'. Fear could 'freeze solid in you' or an incident experienced could 'plague you for weeks'. Communications with colleagues could mean they felt they were 'struggling against a brick wall' or were 'between a rock and a hard place'. In their first year following qualification, they learned the impor-tance of 'putting the ball into play' to bring about changes; 'keeping your eye on things', of making 'on-the-spot decisions' and 'floating ideas' so they could 'move things forward'. Sharing these emotions through using metaphors helped them to empathise with common experiences and benefit from peer support – a key learning resource that might help to change their understandings of their practice.

Emotional intelligence

We have emphasised the learning and benefits to be gained from sharing our emotional experiences with others and engaging in reflective activities. Like Duke (2004:160), you may have discovered the power of reflection: 'the excitement and compelling nature of understanding something new or afresh, the richness of coming to know yourself'. We know reflection is used in nurse education since, as well as technical expertise based on evidence and organisational and management skills, nurses require self-awareness, motivation, self-regulation, empathy and skilfulness in relationships in order to practise effectively. These are the competencies that lie at the heart of what is called emotional intelligence and are essential for any situation where the focus is on interaction with others (people skills).

The notion of emotional intelligence was presented by Salovey and Mayer (1990) and measured using the abilities model, consisting of four general abilities: the ability to recog-nise emotions (in oneself and others), to use emotions to facilitate thinking, to understand the complexities and subtleties of emotions and how they interrelate, and, finally, to manage emotions positively (Riggio and Reichman, 2008). Emotional intelligence was popularised by Goleman (1998), who suggested that those with higher emotional intelligence will be more successful at work and in their personal lives because of their high degree of self-awareness and ability to use emotional experiences to manage relationships more effectively and guide their behaviour. This was seen as particularly relevant for nurses as they need to pay special attention to the emotional cues of others, listen well, and respond to the needs of a variety of other people – patients, relatives and colleagues. Freshwater and Stickley (2004: 93) underline this, reminding us that whilst we need to think rationally when undertaking technical nursing skills we also need to 'intuitively sense the needs and emotions of the person at the receiving end'. Developing emotional intelligence is therefore important not only in terms of the individual but also for organisations as it will affect the potential for teamwork, empowerment, creativity, patterns of communication, flexibility and the acceptance of diversity. It will have an effect on the ways in which we work with individual patients and their families and also on the ways we work with colleagues. In their work on leadership, Riggio and Reichman (2008) highlight the importance of going beyond the emotional skills approach since emotional intelligence also includes the ways in which emotions inform mental processing. They suggested the notion of social intelligence was more apt since it included within it 'the ability to express oneself in social interactions, the ability to "read" and understand different social situations, knowledge of social roles, norms and scripts, interpersonal problem-solving skills and social role-playing skills' (page 171). They presented an integrative model, which, they argued, contained the key emotional and social skills necessary for effective interactions and leadership.

It is not surprising therefore that there has been a great deal of interest around the notion of emotional intelligence in nursing, although Freshwater and Stickley (2004:91) question the uncritical and unthinking application of it within nursing curricula, without 'fully grasping the entirety of its meaning and application'. They noted the importance of interdependence of rational and emotional intelligence and suggested that much more needs to be done to promote stronger links between the two domains. They stressed the importance of helping students throughout the curriculum to engage in learning that transforms or changes practice (in other words, 'transformatory learning'). They suggested a range of activities that they consider to be useful for this, such as self-inquiry, reflective discussion and writing, supportive supervision and mentorship, service user involvement in the planning and delivery of the course, and the use of art, drama, music, film and poetry. It might be helpful for you to consider what resources you have available to you and assess what helps you most in your emotional and social development, the growth of personal strengths and effective ways of responding not only to patients and their relatives but also your colleagues.

It is said that emotional competencies can be cultivated with the right practice if there is readiness to learn, motivation, effective support and clear, honest feedback and guidance. The importance of good role modelling cannot be overestimated. Noddings (2002), an educator and philosopher, discusses this in relation to the notion of developing ethical caring. She goes so far as to claim that we are responsible for the development of every person we encounter, indicating 'How I treat you may bring out the best and worst in you. How you behave may provide a model for me to grow and become better than I am. Whether I can become and remain a caring person – one who enters regularly in caring relations – depends in large part on how you respond to me' (page 15). The impact of the individual mentor on student experience should therefore not be underestimated.

A trusting and supportive learning environment is important for everyone. Opportunities for learning can come from dialogue with critical friends and clinical supervisors. Duke (2004:147), an experienced practitioner, also found it helpful to look for other strategies that helped her explore the meaning of her practice experiences as she describes how at times she became 'stuck in the reflective cycle'. She used poetry, metaphor and concept mapping to broaden and develop her skills. As we have seen, looking more closely at the way you describe your practice experience, e.g. by looking at the meaning of the metaphors you are using, may help you to discover more about yourself and the way you respond emotionally to practice situations.

To think about

We have described the usefulness of metaphors in helping us to understand both ourselves and others and to increase our emotional intelligence. We hope that what you have read will act as an impetus for you to continue to find ways of increasing this and of recognising the impact it has on your ability to care both for yourself and for others. You will find that changes will occur in the ways you both think about caring and act in the future as a result of learning from your emotions. It might be useful to ask yourself the following questions:

+ Are you able to identify the various forms of support and resources that help you most?
+ Have you considered a range of strategies, such as the use of analysis of metaphors or the use of creative approaches such as poetry or drama, to expand your knowledge of self and others?
+ Can you think of ways in which you changed (perhaps in the way in which you make judgements of situations and people or act) as a result of any reflective activity you have engaged in?
+ Has your learning about yourself resulted in some form of emancipation and transformation? In other words, has it freed you from ways of thinking and behaving that were not useful and increased your ability to cope with new or challenging situations in practice?

Reflecting on our possible selves

Whilst we have indicated the importance of being self-aware and highlighted some of the ways we might achieve this, we need to take into account that this journey is not straightforward and never ends as we don't remain static but change from day to day. Sometimes we feel 'spot on' and any problems encountered seem easily solved. However, all of us sometimes feel 'in the pits' and everything seems a struggle. We have different perceptions of ourselves and our capabilities at those times. How we view ourselves at any one particular time depends on what has happened before and what we believe is likely to occur in the future.

Markus and Nurius (1986) described the influence of our 'possible selves', suggesting that when we look at ourselves we make judgements of our value and worth, by taking account of a range of possible selves – what I was like, what I am like and what I might be like in the future. The importance of this is that it emphasises the fact that past and future possible selves (both negative and positive) can exert an influence on our present behaviour and feelings. 'Possible selves represent individuals' ideas of what they might become, what they would like to become and what they are afraid of becoming' (Markus and Nurius, 1986:954).

Using this notion, it is useful to consider the impact on patient or carer perhaps of the fear of an unknown future when faced with long-term or life-threatening conditions. For example, parents of a child with severe disabilities might grieve for the child who 'might have been' and also be anxious about what they as parents might have to become.

'Possible selves' are important as they can act as motivating factors for our behaviour (influencing approaches and avoidance strategies). For example, a student who finds calculations difficult and is frightened of looking foolish might try to avoid assisting with the administration of medications. Rationally, there is no need to feel foolish because we all find some aspects of our work easier than others and the fear that we might have of others discovering our 'deficiencies' might lead to us missing out on an opportunity to learn.

The mixture of perceptions of 'possible selves' is relevant to all of us , particularly at a time of personal or professional change. Reflection can help you in that any ambiguities, tensions and judgements associated with changing self-image and therefore self-esteem can be accessed and utilised to influence the way you think about yourself. We often fear the worst about ourselves, and recognising irrational fears and building up our self-confidence are important. You may find that if you keep a personal diary in which you reflect honestly on your experiences, you can uncover the range of images and irrational thoughts you have about yourself.

Katrina found her first job in a nursing home following registration quite challenging. Read her entry in a reflective journal and think about how the emotions related to her 'possible selves' influenced her self-concept and self-esteem.

Case Study 6.4

'It was only my third shift working at the nursing home. I was on early shift and I was still not used to the routine and the residents' names. Upon arriving at work, I was horrified to discover that the charge nurse (my preceptor) had just phoned in sick and I was to be the only qualified nurse on duty with three health-care assistants. The night staff gave a quick handover to us all, most of the names meant nothing to me, I couldn't put a face to a name. Instead of listening at handover, I felt myself shift into thinking about doing the drugs myself. Then on to emergency situations, there was no resuscitation team here. Hospital seems to be very safe, there are always plenty of people to ask. Here I felt isolated. I questioned my first aid skills and wished that I had done a first aid course; perhaps I'd feel more confident now.

The night staff left and the keys were passed on to me. Those all-important keys. I had a strong feeling of nausea. I allocated the work and we started to get the residents up, working as quickly as we could. I was constantly thinking to myself, "Please don't let anything happen, I'm just not ready." I felt as though I needed more time. At break I just couldn't eat anything, I felt sick and on edge. The shift passed quickly without any incidents and when the late-duty staff nurse came on, I felt relieved and it was with great joy that I passed those keys over to him. I felt as if a ton had been lifted off my back.

Later, I reflected on my day and I felt angry that I could be left without knowing the residents or the routine. But after all, the health-care assistants knew them well. My charge nurse could not help being ill and should anything have occurred, I'm sure common sense would have taken over. I felt really isolated and have realised that nursing homes are now not the easy option that they are portrayed to be but I know I am capable of coping.'

Compare your considerations with ours

Katrina's story provides a powerful image of the impact of a trajectory (journey) of anxiety throughout a shift as she felt the need to prove herself capable and sensed her inadequacies. We can see that her anxiety mounts as the story unfolds until the keys are taken away and the weight of responsibility lifts. She then questions her response as to who was to blame for the circumstances and reassures herself with the knowledge that nothing did go wrong, and if it had, it would probably have been OK anyway.

The telling of the story led to a reassessment of what she perceived she was like. Retelling how she performed in an extremely stressful situation helped her to articulate how she managed to survive, in spite of an early negative view of her own ability that affected her badly. Telling the story had the potential of helping her to overcome her anxieties by making her more aware of her capabilities. It was a story about overcoming adversity and building up her confidence in her ability.

We can see how her exploration of her 'possible selves' influenced her. She redefined herself – by considering what she was like in the past when she had support within a hospital setting, what she was like now (her inexperience and lack of familiarity made her doubt her ability) and what she might be like in the future (during the experience she thought it might all go wrong but by the end she was able to be more confident about the way she had coped and what she was capable of in the future).

It is not known whether Katrina reflected on this situation with her preceptor but it is likely that this might have led on to a clear identification of her learning needs (e.g. concerning emergency situations, giving medications, safety aspects, line management responsibilities and referrals) and also for gaining more reassurance concerning the strengths of her performance. It can be seen, however, that simply by telling the story she had begun the process in which a negative self-image was transformed into one in which she was beginning to see herself in a more positive light. If you do keep a reflective diary you will be able to see changes in the way you perceive yourself.

We have seen other evidence of this recognition of the transformation to a 'capable self' through experience (enhanced by positive feedback). A student described how she coped with (i.e. responded to, initiated the procedure for and managed) an unexpected cardiac arrest. She compared this with her previous 'nervous' self, and was confident that she would continue to be more confident and capable in the future.

Time to think back

Caring for yourself means recognising feelings that may be detrimental to you so that you are then able to respond in a useful way. As we have said, if you are overcome with feelings of inadequacy you are likely to give much greater emphasis to deficiencies in your performance than if you have a positive self-image. However, if you articulate your feelings you will be better able to accept and learn from them. Can you recognise the influence of possible selves? As we have seen, they may be accessed through paying attention to your internal conversations or by writing down how you feel about a given situation.

Articulating and accepting our feelings

Carrie, a newly qualified nurse, found that writing down her feelings about a complex situation raised questions that she needed to answer. Read the following account and consider the questions that it might have raised for her.

Case Study 6.5

'Being a qualified staff nurse, you automatically think that the role/title in itself allows you to be knowledgeable, responsible and able to cope with any situation put before you. Not so. Working in intensive care, there are many situations which you (staff nurse) are supposed to deal with efficiently and maturely without letting personal feelings become involved. One incident occurred when I was looking after a sick patient and basically the decision was made to turn off all the life support. Simple? No, I felt as if I couldn't, wouldn't, be able to. After all, I'm only me, young enough to be this patient's daughter. Yet I was advising his wife, comforting the other relatives and nursing this dying patient in a very mature, responsible, staff nurse way. All the time I simply wanted to say - stop! Try again with this patient - don't let him die, as I can't handle this! Yet as a staff nurse you have to, regardless of your feelings or the person you are. Anyway the shift ended, relatives comforted, paperwork sorted, patient continuously nursed until "his final hour".

I've been told that, in time, you learn to accept it, accept situations more effectively and eventually go home thinking, "I've done a good job today." But that comes with experience. I'll let you know.'

Compare your considerations with ours

+ Is it rational for Carrie to think that 'being a qualified staff nurse, you automatically think that the role/title in itself allows you to be knowledgeable, responsible and able to cope with any situation put before you'?

+ Is she right in thinking that as a staff nurse you should be able to cope with situations without letting personal feelings become involved?

Carrie seems to be questioning whether she is mature enough to cope with the situation. Carrie should ask herself whether she has learned to manage her feelings about death. She might also ask herself to think about what constitutes doing a good job. We think she has unrealistic expectations of what might be expected of her as a newly qualified staff nurse. This notion of a perfect 'possible self' may have begun as a student. She feels she is 'acting' a staff nurse role but her emotions have overtaken her.

The significance of Carrie's story appears to lie in her reaction to the decision to turn off a life support machine and the action of doing so. There is no debate, however, over whether this is right or wrong for the patient (this would have been a team and family decision) but she concentrates on how the action affects her. She appears to be concerned that she has felt ill-equipped to deal with the event because of her inexperience and also personal misgivings - she doesn't want the patient to die. However, she is reinforcing her view that she has overtly supported the decision, by letting the routine take over and acting in a 'staff nurse way' by 'comforting the relatives' and providing care until the 'final hour'.

Carrie is viewing the decision from a personal viewpoint. It appears that she is finding it difficult to deal with the finality associated with the decision. She is indicating that she is unable to be objective and detached in a situation like this (which to her would be a sign of having 'done a good job') and is presenting an image of herself as young, emotional and inexperienced. This is reinforced by making comparisons of the patient as parent and herself as a child. At the end, however, there is an element of doubt that these feelings will continue and the possibility that there will be changes with experience is raised. However, when she reviews the situation with help she might be able to look at the reasons for her fears, e.g. her own or feared losses or death.

Carrie has used the story as a means of expressing her emotional feelings yet to be resolved. Transformatory learning from the situation could have taken place through engaging in various strategies such as using her story as a focus for discussion during pre-ceptorship supervision. Talking this situation over with somebody else, particularly if she had written it down in such detail, would help her think again about her strengths and areas for further development. She could also question whether a caring nurse can remain so whilst being part of 'calculated and detached' decisions. It would seem that in managing her emotions (emotional labour) and putting the needs of the patients and family first, she was fulfilling a caring role.

Accepting our shadow side

Like Carrie, we are all fearful and upset at times and may also experience other feelings such as anger, annoyance, envy, competition, indignation, antagonism and bitterness. We all have a tendency to display what the psychoanalyst Jung (1966) called our 'shadow side'. However, he believed that it was important to find out about, accept and learn from this because of all the potential it has for personal growth. Smith (2004) seems to illustrate this through the work of Noddings, who claims that 'ethical' caring does have to be summoned to overcome such feelings.

> 'The "I ought" arises but encounters conflict: An inner voice grumbles, "I ought but I don't want to," or "Why should I respond?" or "This guy deserves to suffer, so why should I help?" On these occasions we need not turn to a principle; more effectively we turn to our memories of caring and being cared for and a picture or ideal of ourselves as carers . . . Ethical caring's great contribution is to guide action long enough for natural caring to be restored and for people once again to interact with mutual and spontane-ous regard.' (Noddings 1998:187)

Consider the following incident written by Maylin, a second-year student nurse, and think about whether you have experienced similar feelings.

Case Study 6.6

'We visited Dawn, suffering from terminal cancer, in her home. During the visit we were to help her out of bed and put on a TENS machine to relieve the pain. I started to help my mentor put the machine on. To Dawn everything we did was "totally wrong and in the wrong bloody order".

Afterwards we discussed the visit and my mentor said that Dawn had been visited by another community nurse for months and probably didn't like the change. At the time of the incident I felt quite annoyed and frustrated at Dawn's attitude. When I had time to think about it, I felt disgusted with myself since she was in a lot of pain and probably did not have long to live. The most demanding thing was to hide my anger and, although I did not say anything to her, I think that she might have realised that we were both annoyed at her.

I think that this is important to reflect on since it showed me that sometimes it can be very difficult to cover up your feelings and care for someone. I thought that Dawn had made me feel angry and frustrated as nothing we did seemed right. However, as my mentor pointed out, Dawn might have been using angry behaviour to cover up her fear and feelings of insecurity. This helped me to realise that if I get the "wrong feelings" about a patient, a useful coping mechanism might be to accept that we don't really know what is going on in a patient's life.'

So-called negative emotions we feel are often not openly discussed and critically explored. Perhaps this is so especially in our place of work, but that does not mean they are not present. As we saw in Chapter 3, angry patients, those who are perceived as behaving 'badly' or are 'ungrateful' and 'demanding', can be unpopular with nurses and this can affect the care they receive. It is relatively easy to feel compassionate when confronted directly with other people's suffering, but we can feel threatened and disillusioned when faced with an angry patient or relative, because when someone gets angry with us we might get angry in return. We need to acknowledge and manage this. Emotions become threatening the moment they threaten to disrupt our calm and our emotional balance. Somehow we have to distance ourselves from the heat of the drama and find a way of rebalancing.

We may learn a lot about ourselves by reflecting on aspects of patients' behaviour that we find most difficult. This calls for a sort of detective work. It requires self-awareness, such as finding out why, how and when we are at our most vulnerable since different experiences and people affect us all in different ways. Acknowledging what irritates, hurts or annoys us most about other people has the potential to help us to have a greater insight into our personal shadow side, which can otherwise remain hidden. This means that when the patient's behaviour is difficult for us to address we do not see ourselves as a victim, nor do we view ourselves as superior.

Emotions and the therapeutic relationship

We chose the title of this chapter 'Transformative learning – being and becoming' because we wanted to stress the importance of learning to understand our emotional responses and the ways in which they can influence how we relate to others, particularly in terms of establishing and maintaining therapeutic relationships. In mental health nursing such relationships are often seen as the primary interventions but they are important in all areas of nursing occurring alongside other, perhaps more physical, interventions. We have seen that it is often the more intimate interventions such as helping someone with their hygiene, feeding or pain relief that become vehicles through which relationships can be established, trust built up and compassionate care shown. Sadly, it is the neglect of meeting fundamental patient needs, which provide these important opportunities, that have been the focus of many complaints about poor-quality care (e.g. Francis, 2010). How we maintain a culture in which compassion in care can be fostered and supported is vital particularly as practice extends further into the previous domains of medical practice and nurses have to cope with the impact of major advances in technological changes and interventions (Youngson, 2008). Foster and Hawkins (2005) highlight the complexity in terms of knowledge and skills required in building up therapeutic relationships, seeing practice as a major source of learning about these. However, because identification and assessment of therapeutic skills are easily missed or taken for granted within practice these authors set out a 'performance of understanding tool' as a useful method (page 701).

We know that skilled practitioners can play an important part in identifying and explaining the nature of effective relationships and techniques that may help establish these. Liz is a practitioner and researcher working in chest medicine. Using a skilled technique that may be more familiar to nurses working with people with mental health problems, she described her work with Thomas.

Case study 6.7

'Over the last 10 years I have used cognitive behavioural therapy (CBT) skills to develop more effective relationships with patients. It is very important to try to understand what the patient is experiencing. One of the fundamental principles of CBT is that what patients think affects how they feel, what they do and the physical symptoms they experience. The CBT framework enables both the patient and me to make sense of their complex problems and allows us to develop an individual treatment plan together. Thomas has a very severe chronic obstructive pulmonary disease and was experiencing terrible panic attacks. We discussed what triggered these attacks and, how this affected his physical symptoms, what he thought, how he felt and how he coped with them. The panic attacks, it emerged, came on when he exerted himself. He became so breathless he thought he was going to die. Obviously he was very frightened when this happened. To cope he would avoid activity if possible and became very deconditioned and housebound. I summarised what he said to ensure I had captured exactly what he had told me. He agreed I had and said he felt I had been the only person to really take an interest in what he was experiencing. That alone made him feel better and this helped develop a very therapeutic relationship between us. We were then in a much better position to develop coping strategies that would improve the panic attacks. Collaboratively we identified techniques including distraction and building up his activities by breaking them down into small steps. He realised that avoiding activity was actually contributing to his difficulties. His panic attacks disappeared completely.'

It seems evident that through the use of CBT, Liz had the opportunity to focus on Thomas as a person. She engaged in what has been described as the 'therapeutic use of self' by effective communication – she listened and she summarised Thomas's experiences. Because of her obvious interest, they established a relationship of trust so that together they were then able to consider a plan for a successful outcome. The story shows the importance of establishing therapeutic relationships in order to deliver skilled practice. In other words, it is the 'being' as well as the 'doing'. In addition, the development of nursing as a profession is dependent on nurses such as Liz sharing her expertise not only by role modelling but also by sharing her knowledge with wider audiences.

Summary

In this chapter we have focused on what it means to be self-aware. We used examples from practice to discuss how reflection can increase our self-awareness and considered the ways in which we might be analytical about ourselves by using metaphors and images to help us understand more about ourselves and others. We also explored the notion of emotional intelligence and its place in our professional development, including competencies such as self-awareness, motivation, self-regulation, empathy and skilfulness in relationships. We stressed the importance of finding ways of developing these aspects if we are to maintain and enhance caring approaches and establishing relationships that are therapeutic and are more likely to lead to successful outcomes.

We emphasised the role of reflection in increasing our self-awareness. When a strong emotional reaction has occurred it is important to reflect on the situation after the event, away from what Eraut (1994) describes as the 'hot action' where responses and demands in practice can be quite problematic. Sometimes our reflections can be the result of a sudden 'penny dropping' when our understanding takes on a new meaning or we are able to synthesise or integrate our learning experiences. We have also learned that reflection helps us uncover other important influences on our self-image; the impact of our beliefs about how we were in the past or might be in the future and what we are like now (the notion of our 'possible selves'). Recognising ourselves as changing and developing leads to our realising the importance of understanding our ontological knowledge (what we 'are' – our 'being') as well as our epistemological knowledge (what we 'know').

Looking forward

Caring for ourselves is important if we are to fulfil our potential and be caring towards others. A better understanding of what makes us stressed and how we might manage this will help us to learn how to take better care of ourselves and develop emotional resilience to overcome some of the challenges we face. In the next chapter we will consider this and also discuss how consideration of our strengths and resources can help us achieve our goals.

Activity

This activity is designed for students but qualified staff could suggest it as a way of helping students consider their personal professional development as follows:-.

Next time you begin a practice, record or write down your feelings about yourself – how you felt at the end of the first week (no holds barred – it's for your eyes only). Do it again halfway through, and at the very end of the placement review once more how you feel about yourself. Listen to or read your entries and see what you can learn about yourself in relation to past, present and your future possible nursing self.

Caring indicators

1. Learning from reflecting on the emotional aspects of practice; the positive and the negative

2. Paying attention to, accepting and responding to, emotional cues in self and others

3. Acknowledging and managing our 'shadow side', emotions that disrupt our calm and emotional balance, by acknowledging the ethical demand of caring

4. Having the ability to use a variety of reflective techniques and creative strategies to help transform practice

5. Developing emotional and social intelligence including competencies of self-awareness, motivation, self-regulation, empathy and skilfulness in relationships

6. Promoting and developing positive self-concept to increase emotional and physical health and resilience

7. Recognising that what we may think we might be like in the future (our 'possible selves') can be either motivational or based on hidden fears

8. Becoming increasingly aware of and acknowledging our capabilities and our areas for further development

9. Establishing therapeutic relationships as a basis for implementing change

10. Sharing knowledge and expertise with colleagues and wider audiences

References

Atkins, S (2004) Developing underlying skills in the move towards reflective practice. In Bulman, C and Schutz, S (eds) *Reflective Practice in Nursing*. Oxford: Blackwell.

Berne, E (1968) *Games People Play*. Harmondsworth: Penguin.

Duke, S (2004) When reflection becomes a cul-de-sac: strategies to find the focus and move on. In Bulman C and Schutz S (eds) *Reflective Practice in Nursing*. Oxford: Blackwell.

Eraut, M (1994) *Developing Professional Knowledge and Competence*. London: Falmer Press.

Francis, R (2010) Independent Inquiry into care provided by Mid-Staffordshire NHS Foundation Trust January 2005–March 2009. London: Stationery Office.

Foster, T and Hawkins, J (2005) The therapeutic relationship: dead or merely impeded by technology. *British Journal of Nursing* **14**,13, 698–702.

Freshwater, D and Stickley, T (2004) The heart of the art: emotional intelligence in nurse education. *Nursing Inquiry* **11**, 91–98.

Gibbs, G (1988) *Learning and Doing: A Guide to Teaching and Learning Methods*. Oxford: Oxford Polytechnic.

Goleman, D (1995) *Emotional Intelligence*. London: Bloomsbury Publishing.

Goleman, D (1998) *Working with Emotional Intelligence*. London: Bloomsbury Publishing.

Graham, H (1995) *Mental Imagery in Health Care: An introduction to therapeutic practice*. London: Chapman & Hall.

Johns, C (2000) *Becoming a Reflective Practitioner: A reflective and holistic approach to clinical nursing practice development and clinical supervision.* Oxford: Blackwell Science.

Johnson, J (1996) *A Dialectical Examination of Nursing Art.* In Kenney, J (ed) *Philosophical and Theoretical Perspectives for Advanced Nursing Practice.* London: Jones & Barlett Publishers.

Jung, C (1966) *Modern Man in Search of a Soul.* London: Routledge & Kegan Paul.

Kozier, B, Erb, G, Berman, A, Snyder, S, Lake, R and Harvey, S (2008) *Fundamentals of Nursing: Concepts, Process and Practice.* Harlow: Pearson Education.

Madjar, I and Walton, J (1999) *Nursing and the Experience of Illness: Phenomenology in practice.* London and New York: Routledge.

Markus, H and Nurius, P (1986) Possible selves. *American Psychologist* **41**, 954-969.

McQueen, A (2004) Emotional intelligence in nursing work. *Journal of Advanced Nursing* **47**, 101-108.

Noddings, N (2002) Educating moral people: a caring alternative to character education. New York; Teachers College Press.

Riggio, R and Reichard, R (2008) The emotional and social intelligences of effective leadership. *Journal of Managerial Psychology* **23**, 2, 169-185.

Salovey, P and Mayer, J (1990) 'Emotional intelligence', *Imagination, Cognition and Personality,* **9**, 185-211.

Orbach, S (1999) *Towards Emotional Literacy.* London: Virago.

Smith, A (2003) *Learning about Reflection.* PhD thesis, Northumbria University, Newcastle upon Tyne.

Smith, M K (2004) Nel Noddings, The ethics of care and education. *The Encyclopaedia of Informal Education* Available at: **www.infed.org/thinkers/noddings.htm.** (last accessed 15/05/2012).

Sontag, S (1991) *Illness as Metaphor.* London: Penguin.

Stevens, R (1996) *Understanding the Self.* London: Sage.

Thompson, N (2002) *People Skills.* Basingstoke: Palgrave Macmillan.

Thompson, N (2003) *Communication and Language.* Basingstoke: Palgrave Macmillan.

Watson, J (1999) *Postmodern Nursing and Beyond.* London: Churchill Livingstone.

Wetherall, M and Maybin, J (1996) The distributed self: a social constructionist perspective. In Stevens, R (ed) *Understanding the Self.* London: Sage.

Youngson, R (2008) *Compassion in health care* . NHS Confederation Futures debates. Available at: **www.nhsconfed.org/Publications/Pages/Compassion-in-healthcare.aspx** (last accessed 17/03/2012).

Chapter 7
Promoting a culture of caring

LEARNING OBJECTIVES

By the end of this chapter you should have an understanding of:

1. The importance of professional responsibilities in creating and maintaining a culture of caring

2. Ways of recognising, avoiding and managing stress so we can increase our emotional resilience and that of patients, colleagues and carers

3. The value of building on strengths and resources, e.g. using a solution-focused approach and using supportive networks effectively

4. Ways in which we can extend our ability to care for ourselves and others through utilising creative and innovative approaches

5. The importance of providing a culture of caring, free from discrimination, harassment and bullying

Introduction

As we have found, although stress is a part of everyday practice, the ability of some students and qualified nurses to care is diminished if they become overwhelmed with personal and professional issues, including unrealistic expectations of themselves. However, individual reactions to stress are also influenced by the culture in which nurses provide care and will subsequently have an impact on the quality of that care provided for patients. If staff feel unsupported and there is evidence of low staff morale, this may be reflected in elevated absence and sickness rates (Francis, 2010).

Belonging to an effective team in the workplace, within a clear support system, will provide positive and nurturing professional relationships and is likely to promote a culture necessary for the development and maintenance of emotional resilience. This means that individuals are more likely to cope with and learn from any professional challenges they might face. There is evidence that emotional resilience is more than purely an inherent trait or set of individual skills but is the result of the interaction between individual, acquired coping skills, the immediate environment and the broader social, cultural and political context (Brigham and Smith, 2008). Wilkin and Slevin (2004:57), discussing the influence of the team in providing a supportive network in critical care units, highlight the importance of communication, teamwork and mutual support: 'The participants considered working closely with and supporting colleagues as an important element. Teamwork, being there, timeliness in the provision of emotional support and feedback were seen as being important to the participants.'

Effective and engaging managers can provide guidance, frameworks, policies and developmental opportunities that help to ensure the provision of quality care so that staff are supported and enabled to reach their potential. They therefore have an important role to play in motivating and encouraging staff. This tangible support is essential if nurses and all health-care staff are to feel their work is recognised and valued. There are interesting debates concerning the notion of 'distributed' leadership, which means that decision making and accountability are devolved as closely as possible to the frontline of clinical practice. Turnbull James (2011:18) sums up its importance for everyone engaged in care:

'The healthcare context requires people who do not identify with being a leader to engage in leadership. Leadership must be exercised across shifts 24/7 and reach to every individual: good practice can be destroyed by one person who fails to see themselves as able to exercise leadership, as required to promote organisational change, or who leaves something undone or unsaid because someone else is supposed to be in charge. The NHS needs people to think of themselves as leaders, not because they are personally exceptional, senior or inspirational to others, but because they can see what needs doing and can work with others to do it.'

Ensuring high standards of care is therefore the responsibility of all who work within an organisation, but this work may be very demanding. Knowledge of how we develop our own particular positive coping mechanisms will help us to learn how to take better care of ourselves. If we do so, we will be more competent in caring for others and will have satisfaction in a job well done, which in turn can increase our self-esteem. However, Goleman (1999) says that 'empathy distress' is common for those who are in the helping professions, as they continuously have to cope in extreme circumstances and may have to deal with people in unpleasant moods. We therefore have to learn to be emotionally competent and not only aware of our feelings but also be capable of not becoming weighed down by resentment, disillusionment and antagonism, all of which can lead to feelings of failure and guilt. We saw in Chapter 3 how certain people can cause particular problems for staff and may become 'unpopular' patients causing feelings of frustration, anger and resentment and this can adversely affect the quality of the care they receive. For example, progressive deterioration in relationships between patients and staff (which can occur with patients who repeatedly attempt suicide and eventually do so in spite of multiple and intensive interventions) has been described as malignant alienation (Watts and Morgan, 1994). A culture of mutual support and trust is needed to gain an understanding of why this occurs and safe ways for staff to express negative emotions need to be established.

The individual as part of a caring community

Caring for ourselves is important if we are to fulfil our potential, including finding the most effective ways in which we can care for, and work effectively with, others. A better understanding of what makes us stressed and how we might manage this will help us to learn how to take better care of ourselves and develop emotional resilience to overcome some of the challenges we face.

Do you ever go home from your work placement feeling absolutely exhausted emotionally as well as physically? Every nurse, whatever her or his level of experience, encounters stress. This can be a great motivator but it can also have an adverse impact. There are indicators of the beneficial aspects of stress (eustress), such as speedier reaction times and the ability to focus attention on the specific situation. If we are in distress, however, there are negative indicators such as lack of self-esteem, short temper, negative attitudes, and coping mechanisms that may cause us harm, for example smoking and drinking. Stress is a subjective experience arising from individual perceptions and there are many perceived sources (Kozier et al., 2008).

When we are overwhelmed with everyday 'busyness' and don't give ourselves time and space for renewal, we can experience all the signs and symptoms of stress. Covey (1999:287) used the following story to illustrate this:

> 'Suppose you were to come across someone in a wood working feverishly to saw down a tree. "What are you doing?" you ask.
>
> "Can't you see?" comes the impatient reply. "I'm sawing down this tree."
>
> "You look exhausted!" you exclaim. "How long have you been at it?"
>
> "Over five hours." he returns, "and I'm beat! This is hard work."
>
> "Well, why don't you take a break for a few minutes and sharpen that saw?" you inquire. "I'm sure it would go a lot faster."
>
> "I don't have time to sharpen the saw," the man says emphatically, "I'm too busy sawing."'

We often feel too busy to stop but may realise that this is not an effective way of trying to cope with situations. We were reminded of this by a group of ward managers who were engaged in a series of group reflective sessions so that they could share experiences and learn from and support each other. During a winter bed crisis when they were extremely busy, we suggested that they might want to cancel the next session. Back came the reply, 'It's when we're so busy that we need it most.'

Work stress, and its effects, is a serious health issue. As you may have learned in your study of its effects on patients, stress can have severe physical, psychological, social and spiritual effects and many illnesses are either caused or aggravated by stress. In addition Wicks (2006:4) suggests that 'the pressure that results from the reaching out to others in need is a constant and continuous reality in medicine, nursing and allied health' and leads to what he describes as secondary stress. Other factors such as colleague relationships, limited resources, organisational change and pressures also play an important part (Edward and Hercelinskyj, 2007).

In earlier chapters we have referred to the severe and cumulative stress brought about by emotional or physical exhaustion, which can lead to a complex syndrome known as 'burn-out' or compassion fatigue. This is found in people who work in numerous public service occupations including nursing. Signs of burn-out include chronic fatigue and exhaustion, anger, cynicism, negativity, depression, feelings of helplessness and hopelessness and physical effects such as insomnia, headaches, weight loss or gain. There are also reports of an increased likelihood of risk taking (Edward and Hercelinskyj, 2007).

Goleman (1999:288) claims that only a few organisations address the degree to which they themselves create stress and more usually blame the victims of burn-out as if it were entirely the individuals' defect. He cites a study to make his point about the relationship between burn-out amongst nurses and patient satisfaction. 'In a large medical centre, the extent to which nurses on inpatient units had classical burn-out symptoms like cynicism, exhaustion and frustration with working conditions correlated with patients' reports of dissatisfaction with their hospital stay. The more content nurses were with their jobs, the better patients rated their medical care.'

We therefore need to look for ways in which we can prevent undue stress or burn-out happening, not only for ourselves but also because of the effects it will have on the ways in which we are able to care for others and relate to our families, friends and colleagues. In addition, one person's stress seems to be 'catching' and may induce stress in others, leading to what Wicks (2006) describes as 'burn-out contagion' and can therefore have a negative impact on the effective functioning of teams or organisations. An important aspect of leadership is to recognise early indications of this, determine the causes and find ways in which to change the culture into one in which people feel valued and have a shared sense of purpose and which is therefore more conducive to working in harmony and efficiency.

As we saw in Chapter 2, there are positive ways in which difficult situations can be defused. Humour is sometimes used to reduce stress or establish relationships between nurse and patient but Astedt-Kurki and Isola (2001) suggest that humour among staff also helped them to manage difficult issues and situations. 'Humour appeared to relieve the tension within the ward, which resulted in a more liberated and improved working climate' (page 457). Humour, however, has to be used carefully and sensitively. You might have experienced how it can be used as a 'put-down' or in a particularly damaging way, e.g. in jokes based on race, ethnicity, age, gender or sexual orientation.

An extract from Smith's (2003) research study demonstrates how a newly qualified nurse felt belittled by a more experienced colleague:

> 'The senior staff nurse came to me and she said, "X, you didn't do that lady's apex pulse" and I hadn't, I'd forgotten. I sort of went "Well, all right, very sorry" – and she literally told me wherefore and why not in front of the student and the whole bay of sick ladies and I've never felt so humiliated and so annoyed in my whole life actually. And I just said, "I'll do it now." I just forgot – I thought I must have taken someone else to the loo and forgotten to do that one and moved on. And she said, "Well, you know it's very important that you do this because da-da-da . . . " and I said "I know, I **do** know" and as I said, that was in front of a student **and** a bay full of ladies . . . I think she bears a grudge. This is one of the girls who is currently doing the post-registration degree and as soon as she found I'd got it already she said, "Well, how have you already done it?" You go through explaining and she said "Well, it doesn't really matter because you haven't had as much experience as I have . . . " '(page 61)

Experiences such as this can be a sign of a culture in which bullying and horizontal violence are occurring. All nurses need to understand how and why this might occur but managers have a particular responsibility in ensuring that it is prevented through education and anti-bullying and anti-discrimination policies but also in recognising and eliminating it. Freire (1972) uses the term 'horizontal violence' to describe intergroup conflict demonstrated in overt or covert non-physical hostility, which may consist of sabotage, infighting, or scape-goating. He argues that it occurs within a group whose members lack power or autonomy and feel devalued. They then look for someone else to 'oppress'. It can result in the establishment of a culture of negativity in which people are bullied, belittled or criticised in front of others. The notion has since been applied to many organisations and professions including nursing (Farrell, 2005). Horizontal violence is problematic since it adds more to the tension of the work situation and results in damaged self-esteem and loss of confidence. It can become endemic within a culture and lead to stress, low morale and sickness, with individuals leaving the profession. Importantly, it can also affect the quality of care provision.

The NHS Constitution (Department of Health, 2012:10) underpins the obligation for organisations to ensure this does not occur, indicating that staff must:

+ have healthy and safe working conditions and an environment free from harassment, bullying or violence;
+ be treated fairly, equally and free from discrimination;
+ be able to raise an internal grievance and if necessary seek redress, where it is felt that a right has not been upheld.

Developing resilience

There are less likely to be problems associated with stress, even in pressurised situations, if the value or importance of the work is recognised. Ongoing stress is related to how it is perceived by us and by others (Wilkes, 2002). Individuals who see the relevance and value of the work they are undertaking have the ability to 'bounce back' when meeting challenges or adversity and are less likely to experience emotional exhaustion (Glasberg et al., 2007).

The reality and challenges of practice may mean nurses having to come to terms with a working environment that can at times be both rewarding and exhilarating but at other times hostile and difficult. It is easy for our attention to focus on the negative, particularly at the times when we feel physically and emotionally exhausted. For students, this might account for the second year 'dip' and also for the panic just before registration when they are undertaking the final practice placement. This can be a particularly stressful time as they struggle to meet important academic requirements and as the realisation of what it might mean to be a qualified nurse dawns. Knowing that other students experience these 'dips' can help them feel that they are not alone. On the other hand, they may have experienced 'stress contagion' within their peer group when one person's fears and grievances are 'caught' and influence the ways in which all members of the group feel, think and act.

Some ways of thinking appear to block other more positive thoughts and make it difficult for us to move on and overcome negativity. We become overly pessimistic and there is a tendency to blame others for our feelings and situations. It is obvious that in life we may not always be treated fairly and that things can happen that are sad, frustrating, unfair and even disastrous. Whilst it is important to acknowledge the problem and analyse why we are upset, angry or disappointed about a workplace situation, it is not helpful to spend too much time on discussions about who or what was to blame. This can inflame our dissatisfaction so it is better to look for ways in which we can overcome our anxieties, cope with and handle difficult situations.

Abraham (2004) emphasises the value of developing emotional resilience, which he describes as 'flexible optimism'. Instead of engaging in fault-finding, individuals with this are optimistic enough to put difficulties behind them and redirect their attention to positive means of coping. This is not easy to achieve, however.

Consider the case study below and think about how you might help Melanie, a second-year student, overcome the ongoing negative feelings she has about the following event.

Case Study 7.1

'I was asked by a health-care assistant to help her with one of the patients, a large lady who required a hoist in order to be moved or handled. The health-care assistant asked me to help her lift this patient onto the commode without any lifting aids or equipment. Having assessed the situation I knew it was unsafe to lift and so refused to do so without the use of a hoist. Having explained my reasons for not helping, I stated that if she got the appropriate equipment I would certainly assist her.

At first I felt proud that I had been assertive and that I had used my skills of assessment, making a decision relevant to the safety of the three of us. However, the health-care assistant showed her disapproval in front of the patient and other members of staff. After that, I felt she took every opportunity to find fault with me and put me down. I know I made the right decision regarding patient harm and back injuries, but I still feel upset that I had been made to feel an "unpopular nurse" and situations like this when I know I'm doing the right thing but others only want to get the job done quickly really get me down and make me feel like giving it all up.'

Compare your considerations with ours

First of all Melanie would need someone to listen empathetically to what she was saying. You might have identified that it would be important to let her know that you understand and empathise with her by showing acceptance of her feelings, using the skills of paraphrasing, reflecting back and helping her to clarify her concerns and problems. It would be important to acknowledge feelings such as anger and wanting to give up her career.

To help her overcome her distress, we expect you have noted how important it would be to help Melanie to reflect on the positive aspects of the situation, about her caring skills, risk management, and her concern for the physical safety of her colleagues as well as the patient. Another positive aspect would have been recognition of the assertiveness skills she displayed and that she was acting in accordance with the NMC Code (2008). All this will reinforce that she is working well and that she should not 'lose heart' because of this one situation.

The question Melanie might find useful now is to consider what her next actions might be. When not so angry she might feel able to talk things over with the health-care assistant, or she may need the assistance of her mentor or her personal tutor.

If you look back at the above you can see that Melanie might have used two types of coping strategies that have been identified in the literature: problem-focused and emotion-focused (Kozier et al., 2008). Problem-focused coping strategies help by undertaking action that could improve a situation (in this case discussion about why it was so important to move a patient safely). However, Melanie also needed to find ways of relieving her emotional distress by using an emotion-focused strategy (in her case by using a reflective approach which would help her to get things into perspective and reinforce the value of the care she provided).

To think about

Have you ever been in a situation when you have been upset by what a colleague has said to you?

+ How well did you think you managed your feelings; in other words, what coping strategies were you able to use?
+ What resources did you use to help you cope, e.g. people (colleagues, mentor, preceptor, supervisor, personal tutor, friend), or actions related to distraction or relaxation (e.g. physical exercise, meditation, yoga, reading, having a long bath)? Try to be honest about any negative coping strategies you might use such as over-use of alcohol, taking your frustrations out on someone else, e.g. a family member or the cat.
+ What do you need to do in the future to remind yourself of your strengths and to cope with any prolonged negativity such as bearing a grudge?

The solution-focused approach (brief therapy or appreciative approach)

Various approaches have been used to try to get people to consider how to overcome difficulties. Miller and Berg (1995) describe the use of a solution-focused approach in their work, particularly with clients who have a history of alcohol abuse. They make the point that it is not unusual for an individual's strengths to be hidden beneath a mound of negative feelings, such as shame, guilt or disgust. They say that pain is a useful starting point for awareness and reflection but it does not help the solution. 'Pain may get us started, but strengths and resources help us to stay on track and finish the job' (Miller and Berg, 1995:25). It is also evident that many of our patients experience this and may use inappropriate coping strategies. Niall, a student nurse, told us of the frustration he felt in caring for Tyrone, who experienced auditory hallucinations and delusions. Tyrone, frightened by these, found that the only way he felt he could cope was by getting very angry and shouting at the voices until they went away, but also by engaging in alcohol and drug abuse. Changing these ineffective and damaging coping strategies was problematic and required a multi-professional approach, using appropriate resources, in order to help Tyrone to master his problems.

This strategy of focusing on solutions rather than only on problems has been useful in helping many people overcome difficulties by providing a more positive and constructive framework. For example, in Alcoholics Anonymous people are asked to focus on the good parts of the day.

Getting, receiving and reflecting on feedback from others help us to become more aware of our strengths and resources, which can then be used to our advantage in overcoming future problematic situations and combating adverse conditions. Strategies such as effective clinical supervision, mentorship or that undertaken by academic link tutors are therefore essential. Consider how this might work in practice:

Case Study 7.2

Lara was in her final clinical placement, an acute admissions unit, preparing for registration as a qualified staff nurse. She was feeling overwhelmed and asked to see Joanne, her personal guidance tutor. Joanne went to the unit and was concerned to see a tearful and distraught Lara. That day, although the unit was very busy, a decision had been made that Lara should lead a team so that she could work towards the proficiencies she needed in leadership and management skills. Lara said, 'I hope to get a job on this unit when I qualify and the interviews will be coming up soon. I was here before as a second-year student and I loved it so much so I asked to return for my final placement but this morning has been an absolute nightmare.'

Joanne arranged to take her to a quiet place so they would have time to talk through the situation. Lara said, 'I feel I have totally lost my confidence. I'll never be ready in time. How can I be a caring nurse and cope with all of this? I haven't even got the confidence to delegate any more. I feel as if I don't know what I'm doing.'

Joanne listened to Lara's description of a whole series of events that had taken place that morning. Anxious relatives who had been concerned that their father wasn't receiving adequate care, pressure on beds resulting in a rapid turnover of admissions and transfers, junior staff who questioned the way she was delegating responsibilities, and a remark from another member of staff indicating that she would have to work faster if she was to be any use as a staff nurse. Joanne reminded herself that up to now she had not been aware of any problems with Lara's performance. On the contrary, she had received very positive comments from mentors throughout the programme and had always seemed to fit in well with colleagues.

Joanne decided to use a solution-focused approach (adapted from McKergow and Clarke, 2005, with permission) to try to assist Lara to get back on track. In this a number of questions are used to help her move forward.

Think about a 'miracle'

Joanne asked Lara the following question: 'If you were to wake up tomorrow morning and a miracle had happened whilst you'd been asleep and all your problems had gone, what would be the first thing that would be different and who would notice it?'

Lara started to describe herself as a perfect staff nurse who could cope with 'anything that was thrown at her'. She would be a nurse who was very calm, skilled and compassionate, very efficient and quick when undertaking tasks and highly regarded by everyone. Because Joanne wanted Lara to be able to describe this 'miracle' in as much detail as possible, they also looked at the NMC proficiencies and the job description for a junior qualified member of nursing staff. They made a note of what they would add to Lara's initial response to help to describe some of the professionally identified skills needed to reach the 'miracle'.

Lara thought that the first thing that she and then other people would notice would be that 'I would be more together'. Joanne asked her what this 'togetherness' would look like and Lara indicated that she would be calm in the chaos of everyday care and crisis situations and know what things to tackle first. Staff would listen to her and respond without too much moaning and groaning when she delegated. She would then be able to go off duty and relax without worrying all the time about what had happened that day.

Using a scaling question

Joanne then asked Lara to imagine a scale of 0 to 10, with the 'miracle' ranked as a 10 and 0 indicating no understanding or skills about what her image of a qualified nurse should do and be. She asked Lara to consider where she now placed herself on the scale. Lara thought she was at a 5 on the scale.

What has worked in the past and what resources were useful?

Joanne asked Lara to consider how she had reached that point on the scale, considering what strengths, achievements and resources she used. She assisted Lara in identifying what these were. She asked Lara to consider exceptions to the problems; situations when she hadn't panicked but felt in control, even if the unit was very busy. Lara described several situations when emergencies had happened and she felt she had responded well, although she hadn't been in overall charge.

Together they concluded that Lara had a variety of effective skills and resources that she could draw on and develop. For example, Lara had demonstrated that she was patient focused in her care, was very methodical and responsive to acute situations, was highly motivated and had good time-management skills. She wasn't frightened to ask questions and used a range of resources to enhance her learning including observation of good role models, used her reflective skills and written resources such as research articles and policies. Lara noted that in the past she was able to act as if she was calm even though she may have felt quite anxious inside. 'I've watched other people who seem calm,' she said, 'and I've tried to copy them.'

Taking small steps forward

Joanne asked Lara what she could do now to reach a 5.5 or a 6 on the scale. This was achieved by, firstly, looking at her 'miracle' and also reminding herself again of the internal and external resources available to her. In other words, what she had found to work well in the past and why. Joanne then asked Lara to identify something that she could achieve by the following week which was observable, achievable, realistic, specific and measurable. Lara said that she would try not to show how panicky she felt inside; instead she would act in a calm manner. She would do this by continuing to work towards the leadership and management proficiencies (related to delegating tasks) but take particular notice of when she was successful in maintaining a calm manner and when she was unable to do this and why. She would ask her mentor to give her specific feedback.

Lara also remembered that one of her resources in the past had been the keeping of a personal reflective diary. She thought this was a good way of monitoring her progress if she was honest and documented when she felt calm and self-assured as well as situations where she might have displayed lack of confidence and anxiety. She then needed to analyse her thoughts, feelings and behaviour and learn from her successes. Joanne then reminded her that key to her progress would be to do more of what works well, e.g. she might try giving a rationale to staff of why she had delegated in a particular way. If she found that this approach was time-consuming and led to arguments, she could leave this unsuccessful method and try a different approach.

Moving on up the scale

Lara and Joanne discussed the rationale for, and the implications of, continuing the solution-focused approach with Lara's mentor, who agreed to help. Her mentor pointed out that Lara wouldn't have to get to a 10 by the end of the placement – perhaps 8 or 9 would be more realistic. Nobody was expecting that kind of miracle!

The mentor felt that one of the problems for Lara was that she had had too great an expectation of herself in too short a time and that the solution-focused approach would really help her by breaking down her ultimate target into achievable goals and would help her to appreciate and use her successes along the way.

For Lara this approach was very successful and helped her to gain all of her proficiencies by the end of the placement. In addition, she was enthusiastic about the way this had helped her to prepare for a successful job interview because she had looked so carefully at her detailed 'miracle' image of a staff nurse and her own strengths and resources. She knew what was expected of a qualified nurse and had the confidence and self-esteem to perform well at interview.

Application of the solution-focused approach to patient care

McAllister (2003) sees the solution orientation of this approach as an exciting way forward for nursing in terms of both professional development and care for clients. Whilst the part that problem-solving can play is acknowledged, focusing on what is going right and building on strengths, achievements and capacity can help maximise potential. She explains that during periods of stress, thinking becomes more rigid. As Lara found, it is hard to look beyond the problem. McAllister questions whether the problem-based approach alone, useful though it might be in many ways, is tending to constrain nursing and may also have a negative effect on the client in terms of the balance of power. 'Being the problem-solver works to privilege and illuminate the health carer's actions, whilst the work of being a client, struggling to survive, overcome and maintain resilience is overlooked' (McAllister, 2003:530). The solution-focused approach, with its orientation towards the identification and use of personal strengths, qualities and resources, is therefore well suited to nursing and may help us to articulate the importance of and develop effective, caring approaches in partnership with patients and their families.

To think about

Think of a goal that you would like to achieve over the next few months. Follow the steps in the framework used by Joanne to help Lara to see if a solution-based approach might help you in your development.

+ Ask yourself the 'miracle' question – describe the 'perfect' state you would like to be in.
+ Say where you are now on an imaginary scale from 0 to 10, with the 'miracle' ranked as 10.
+ Write down what strengths, achievements and resources you have used to reach the point where you are now on the scale.
+ Think about what small steps you could take to reach the next point up on the scale. Remind yourself again of the internal and external resources available to you. Think carefully about how you will be able to tell that you have achieved it – in other words, set yourself a realistic and observable goal.
+ Move up the scale by continuing to take a series of small steps. Do more of what works well and if something is not working try something different. You might want to consider at what point you will be satisfied that you have reached your maximum point on the scale, taking into account the stage in your professional development. It might take some time to reach 'perfection' depending on the nature of the goal you set yourself. However, the scaling approach will help you to clarify the direction you need to take and to feel good about the distance you have travelled. It will also help you to remember your strengths and the resources you can use.

How building up our emotional resilience will help us to care

You will remember from Lara's story that her initial lack of confidence led to her feeling inadequate, overwhelmed and therefore not able to think clearly and function as effectively as she might. Using the solution-focused approach to help her identify her strengths, being more aware of her successes and the resources available began to make her think and feel very differently about herself. In other words, she became more emotionally resilient in that she would be more likely in the future to perceive challenges or problems as learning opportunities. According to Tusaie and Dyer (2004:3), resilience is 'a combination of abilities and characteristics that interact dynamically and allow an individual to bounce back, cope successfully and function above the norm in spite of significant stress or adversity'.

As we have found, the management of our emotions has important implications for practice since memory functions best when the mind is calm, influencing our capacity to pay attention and pick up cues (Abraham, 2004). Nurses often refer to the way in which they 'cope' with situations and earlier we described problem-focused and emotion-focused strategies. Using strategies such as the solution-focused approach will help support and develop an individual's strengths and therefore their ability to cope with difficult, new or challenging situations. Coping and resilience are related concepts but coping refers to the thinking and behaviour we use to manage the demands of specific stressful situations whereas resilience refers to an overall or more generalised ability (Campbell-Sills et al., 2006).

An increase in self-awareness can help us to make a more rational judgement of our capabilities and reactions and, if we feel any criticism unjustified, to seek constructive dialogue (Abraham, 2004). We need therefore to learn to apply the same kind of critical analysis to ourselves as we might apply to academic work. Becoming more aware and analytical about our emotional reactions to situations will help us not only to regain equilibrium but also to recognise inappropriate or unhelpful reactions. Jackson et al. (2007:6), however, suggest that nurses need help to do this, by focusing on ways in which personal resilience can be fostered. They identify five main ways for facilitating this: building positive nurturing relationships and networks, maintaining positivity, developing emotional insight, achieving life balance and spirituality, and becoming more reflective.

We can therefore enhance our resilience by engaging in reflective practice and utilising strategies that help us to develop our strengths and focus on solutions to things we find difficult. We can also be helped by receiving positive feedback and encouragement, perhaps through recognising the resources we have. These might be in clinical supervision, preceptorship, mentor and peer group support. We can also build up a network of people who 'nurture' us by giving us support and guidance (which will help us to maintain our motivation and positivity). However, we also have to ensure that we give ourselves time to renew ourselves, achieving what Jackson et al. (2007) call a 'life balance'. We can do this by various methods of relaxation and stress reduction but also by making time for other priorities in our lives such as family and friends. Finding the best balance between work, study, family and social life is sometimes difficult but this is essential if we are to function effectively. The more resilient we are, the more effective we will be as caring nurses.

We should also be aware of the importance of helping to develop resilience in others, including colleagues and patients. This is particularly important in leadership and management but also in ongoing interactions with families and carers. Helping others to become more resilient can be achieved through engaging in support and encouragement but also by working in partnership with them to identify and use the internal and external resources available to them (see Chapter 5).

Caring is using our creativity to find solutions

In the complex and often highly organised world of professional care we may forget how our personal experiences and knowledge may be an important resource. Read the following published story in which Perry (2005:45) describes how she used a creative approach and drew on her own memories as a resource to help calm an extremely restless and agitated 85-year-old man.

Case Study 7.3

'Then I heard him repeat a series of words in a garbled fashion and recognised the words of an old hymn. I began to sing the hymn and immediately he became quiet. The change was instantaneous and profound . . . As long as the hymns were sung the patient rested . . . I loved being his nurse because none of the textbook interventions worked. He required flexible, creative nurses who were not afraid to try the unconventional and who were willing to stay. Large doses of sedation made no difference. Somewhere in the deepest levels of this man's mind our presence through music and just being near him touched him. It was a profound night because all my years of training and education came down to the simple singing of a song and using music to touch his soul.'

For us, the account highlights the artistry of caring. Artists are creative and have the ability to look at things in a different way – they help us to see things in a new light. Perry (2005) noticed the familiar words of a hymn and then used her knowledge of this to find a creative way of communicating with the patient. It is sometimes in everyday ways that we can use our creativity. One of our students recalled a situation that occurred during a visit to a client in the community. He needed his feet soaking but the only bowl available was a washing-up bowl. The qualified nurse decided to leave the foot care for another time but was impressed when the student suggested using a plastic bag to line the bowl so that the care could be implemented there and then. The client was very grateful as, because of the student's creative approach, he was given immediate relief from his discomfort.

To think about

Reflect on the ways in which nurse–patient relationships can become therapeutic and healing by using our creativity.

+ Think of ways in which this occurs in everyday practice – perhaps through humour, shared interests, appropriate self-disclosure, conversations, play, touch and actions.
+ Think of situations that you have seen or perhaps experienced yourself in which 'unusual' caring approaches were used to benefit the patient. They could include, for example, the use of art, poetry, play, music, drama.
+ Do you think we recognise and use and value ourselves as a valuable therapeutic and creative resource?

The artistry of caring can be seen within nurse–patient relationships. McAllister (2003:533) claims that nursing needs to remind itself and others of its uniqueness as a profession because 'it has as its essence the human qualities of nurturance, care, presence and connection'. Work by Dame Cicely Saunders (2002:30), founder of the hospice movement in the UK, reinforces this. She says that it is the very way care is given that can 'reach the most hidden places and that this may be an enabler of a search for spiritual peace'. She describes a male patient with incontinence being reassured by being told that 'it's the disease, not you'. The patient describes how he gradually came to forget 'that silly male pride' because the nurses talked to him all the time they were washing and changing him, undertaking the task with such dignity and care that in the end he said he found that 'he didn't give a damn'. In other words, the nurses transformed a situation that could have been undignified and embarrassing for him (affecting his self-image and self-esteem) into one of acceptance and self-respect.

This is an example of the importance of the artistry of care. When this artistry is missing, it can lead to negative emotions such as distress and loss of hope as seen in Chapter 3, and can detrimentally affect health or the journey to a peaceful death. By articulating and reflecting on the way we give care, we can see the importance of the care we have given. We can use it as a way of reinforcing the value of the relationships we develop with our patients and clients. It is easy to overlook these aspects as important successes, all of which could add to the way in which we are able to see ourselves in a positive light and value what we bring of ourselves to our profession. The more we articulate these aspects, the more we are likely to value ourselves and others will value us too.

Helping patients to draw on and develop their own resources

As we have said, it is often when undertaking perhaps the simplest tasks of nursing that we are able to touch another human being deeply as they struggle for meaning and hope in their life.

Case Study 7.4

'Tom was recovering from an amputation of his right leg. He was very quiet and didn't seem to want to make conversation. He rarely asked for help and, as he was MRSA positive, was isolated in a single room and didn't see many people. I thought that being alone and immobile was what was bothering him. One day, I was helping him to shower and dress (a time-consuming process) when I managed to engage him in conversation. He talked about holidays he had enjoyed in the past but said that now because of his amputation he wouldn't be able to plan another. I didn't feel I could reassure him that holidays were possible because I didn't want to give him false hopes about goals he might not be able to achieve.

When the dressing came off he asked me what the wound was like. I asked him if he would like to see the scar. He refused at first but I offered him a mirror and said that if he couldn't look at it at that time I could take the mirror away again. He then said he wanted to see it and so I placed the mirror in front of him. He sort of yelled at first but I just sat quietly and asked if he wanted the mirror taken away. He didn't. He looked a while longer and then said that it didn't look that bad now that he had seen it. He spoke about a friend of his who had had an amputation during the war in a prisoner-of-war camp without anaesthetic using a meat knife and a saw. He said that if his friend could still go on holiday with one leg then so could he.

He seemed a lot better, and when his wife visited him he asked for a haircut. I couldn't believe the change in his appearance. He looked younger, his eyes were twinkling and he was smiling. He admitted to being quite vain for a "man of his age" and was more worried about how his amputation appeared to people. I was quite wrong to think that he was worried about his mobility. I think that because he was elderly I missed the fact that his appearance would still be very important. I won't forget that lesson.'

This account is important because it reminds us of what we mean by caring. The nurse helped Tom to draw on his own resources through her interactions, and helped him to articulate them and reframe his problem. He overcame his fear of the scar and in doing so was able to make comparisons with his friend's experience and gain a renewed sense of hope and dignity. As a nurse you share precious and important moments with others as they struggle to come to terms with perhaps a long-term or stressful condition, loss, altered body image or even death. Many nurses see the fact that they are able to get so close to others in moments of extreme sadness but also moments of extreme happiness as a great privilege that can be regarded as a spiritual dimension of nursing. Watson (1988) describes this kind of close interaction that takes place between patient and nurse as transpersonal – a spiritual union – one in which deep experience is shared.

Spirituality as a resource in health care

People who belong to a particular faith may be helped to understand and make sense of their lives, and consideration of an individual's religious needs is an important aspect of holistic assessment, whatever their age. Gaining knowledge of, or information about, resources we can use to help people to practise and gain solace from their faith is an important part of a nurse's role. However, we may fail to help many patients if we think only in terms of organised religion. Moss (2002:40) quotes Buber (1957), a Jewish theologian, who once observed that there is nothing like religion 'for hiding the face of God' and highlights the fact that practitioners in health and social care are often faced with clients who are searching for meaning in their lives, a significant spiritual quest. You may have come across patients who have asked you the question 'Why me?' or have shown signs of despair or loss of hope or purpose. We may feel that responding to spiritual concerns like this is not part of our role but Moss (2002:44) reminds us that 'We can no more give a sense of meaning and purpose to someone else than we can eat or breathe for them. But to share that journey with them can help them feel valued; which is the first step to a regaining of purpose and meaning.'

Bash (2004:15) suggests that this spiritual journey is different for everyone:

'But what we can say is that each person formulates his or her own spiritual co-ordinates, sometimes consciously and sometimes not. Spirituality is therefore an elastic, subjective description about a person and about the way they express their humanity.

For some this may be to do with values; for others, an experience of the transcendent. For some it may be to do with personal growth; for others about prayer. The task of the nurse who seeks to engage with a person's spirituality is to engage with that person without presuppositions about what their spirituality may be or what spirituality means to them. 'It will then be that, as the Patients' Charter stipulates, we will respect a person's religious, spiritual and cultural needs at all times.'

Wright (2006) also suggests that meaning, value and hope signify a great deal to people but may be relegated down the list of priorities behind organisational and clinical matters. We can only do this by valuing ourselves and also our colleagues. He discusses work in Scotland, where students of nursing, divinity and medicine came together to explore spirituality and health in their work with people with mental health problems and learning disabilities. 'Our aim is to help professionals develop more whole, more compassionate, more spiritual approaches to care that are integrated into everyday work. But we can only talk seriously about this when we have successfully made this a multidisciplinary approach' (Wright, 2006:25). The author claims that as people learn to experience and understand patients differently so their practice begins to change. Learning together across disciplines is a valuable method of building up team resources and acknowledging the contribution each profession can make.

Summary

In this chapter we have discussed all kinds of demanding situations and pressures that nurses experience, leading to excessive stress. We have highlighted the importance of recognising and managing this and of looking after ourselves and others. If the relevance and value of the work nurses undertake are recognised, by their managers as well as by patients, and they also have the ability to 'bounce back' when meeting challenges or adversity, they will be less likely to be at risk of becoming overwhelmed and experiencing emotional exhaustion. Emotional resilience develops if solutions as well as problems or difficulties are acknowledged and the strengths and resources of oneself and others utilised. Some strengths and resources may be easily overlooked, such as our creativity and the close and 'spiritual' relationships we develop with patients and clients. These all help us to improve the 'artistry' in caring and also help to sustain positive feelings about ourselves. All this needs to be undertaken within a culture in which caring for patients and also for staff is central.

We have also suggested that a solution-focused approach is a beneficial tool, both for our own development and also for use in the development of others including patients/clients and their families. You may have noticed strong parallels between this chapter and Chapter 5 (Creating caring partnerships with service users and their families) because many of the caring indicators useful for helping us as professionals to care for ourselves also help us to care for others and to recognise their needs within the caring process (e.g. through the giving and receiving of positive feedback, feeling valued, knowing and using a range of resources and coping with competing demands). This underlines the importance of understanding more about the nature of caring and valuing caring as the central aspect of nursing as we share with others in our common humanity.

Looking forward

In Chapter 8, we will revisit and integrate the caring indicators which we have uncovered and specified at the end of each chapter. This resource will provide us with an overview of the 'artistry' of a caring nurse.

Activity

Think about personal aspects which you might have but want to develop further. The following framework will help you to take responsibility for your personal and professional development. You may find it useful to write down your answers to the questions which are loosely based on Goleman's (1999:26) personal competency framework. Your answers could form the basis of a personal action plan or a dialogue with your mentor, clinical supervisor or a trusted critical friend.

Are you self-aware?
Give an example of your ability to recognise your emotions and their effects on your performance.

+ Make a list of your strengths and areas for further development.
+ Describe how you feel about yourself in terms of your self-worth and capabilities.

How do you self-regulate – manage your emotions, impulses and resources?

+ Describe a time when you were able to keep disruptive emotions and impulses in check and/or a time you found it difficult.
+ Give an example of a time you've been honest or conscientious in your practice, e.g. admitted a lack of knowledge or skill, truth telling, demonstrated how well you can work with other team members.
+ Give an example of how you have been flexible and/or innovative in your approach to practice.

Are you motivated?

+ Describe ways in which you have improved or worked towards achieving a standard of excellence.
+ Give an example of the way you made use of a learning opportunity the last time you were in practice.
+ Describe how persistent you have been in pursuing goals despite obstacles and set-backs.

Please don't be too hard on yourself but use this as a guide for honest self-development.

Caring indicators

1. Promoting a culture in which team members feel valued and have a shared sense of purpose and responsibility for quality care delivery

2. Developing the artistry of compassionate care through creative and innovative approaches

3. Developing compassionate approaches to care, recognising individual spiritual needs, values and beliefs

4. Helping to provide a culture of caring, free from discrimination, harassment and bullying

5. Leading by example through shared decision making, being accountable for judgements and actions and in enabling others to reach their potential

6. Developing and using supportive resources and networks (e.g. clinical supervision, mentor and preceptorship, peer group support)

7. Recognising and responding to times of particular stress for individuals and groups, e.g. during life transitions and periods of loss and change

8. Recognising the impact of negative coping strategies on self and the care we provide and developing positive coping strategies to deal with stress

8. Being aware of and avoiding 'stress contagion' and negativity, recognising indicators of 'burn-out' in colleagues and the effects it can have on patient care   .

10. Developing positive coping skills in ourselves, colleagues, patients and carers

References

Abraham, R (2004) Emotional competence as antecedent to performance: a contingency framework. *Genetic, Social and General Psychology Monographs* **130**, 117-143.

Astedt-Kurki, P & Isola, A (2001) Humour between nurse and patient, and among staff: analysis of nurses' diaries. *Journal of Advanced Nursing* **35**, (3), 452-458.

Bash, A (2004) Issues in clinical nursing: Spirituality. *Journal of Clinical Nursing* **13**, 11-16.

Brigham, L, Smith, A (2008) *Riding the waves; an exploration of how students undertaking a pre-registration nursing programme develop emotional resilience.* Professional and Practice Based learning, Centre for Excellence in Teaching and Learning (PBPL CETL) project, the Open University.

Campbell-Sills, L, Cohan, S and Stein, M (2006) Relationship of resilience to personality, coping and psychiatric symptoms in young adults. *Behaviour Research and Therapy* **44**, 585-599.

Covey, S (1999) *The Seven Habits of Highly Effective People.* London: Simon & Schuster.

Department of Health (2012) *The NHS Constitution (2012)* Available at: **http://www.dh.gov .uk/en/PublicationsandstatisticsPublications/PublicationsPolicyAndGuidance/ DH_132961** (last accessed 23/04/2012.

Edward, K and Hercelinskyj, G (2007) Burnout in the caring nurse: learning resilient behaviours. *British Journal of Nursing* **16**, 240-242.

Farrell, G (2005) From tall poppies to squashed weeds: why nurses don't pull together more? *Journal of Advanced Nursing* **35**, (1), 26-33.

Francis, R (2010) *Independent Inquiry into care provided by Mid-Staffordshire NHS Foundation Trust January 2005-March 2009*. London: Stationery Office.

Freire, P (1972) *Pedagogy of the oppressed*. Harmondsworth: Penguin.

Glasberg, A, Eriksson, S and Norberg, A (2007) Burnout and 'stress of conscience' among health care personnel. *Journal of Advanced Nursing* **57**, 392-403.

Goleman, D (1999) *Working with Emotional intelligence*. London: Bloomsbury.

Jackson, D, Firtko, A and Edenborough, M (2007) Personal resilience as a strategy for surviving and thriving in the face of workplace adversity: a literature review. *Journal of Advanced Nursing* **60**, 1, 1-9.

Kozier, B, Erb, G, Berman, A, Snyder, S, Lake, R and Harvey, S (2008) *Fundamentals of Nursing: Concepts, process and practice*. Harlow: Pearson Education.

McAllister, M (2003) Doing practice differently: solution-focused nursing. *Journal of Advanced Nursing* **41**, 528-535.

McKergow, M and Clarke, J (2005) *Positive Approaches to Change: Applications of Solutions Focus and Appreciative Inquiry at Work*. Cheltenham: Solutions Books.

Miller, S and Berg, I (1995) *The Miracle Method: A radically new approach to problem drinking*. London: Norton & Company.

Moss, B (2002) Spirituality: a personal view. In Thompson, N (ed) *Loss and Grief*. Basingstoke: Palgrave Macmillan.

NMC (Nursing and Midwifery Council) (2008) *The Code: Standards of conduct, performance and ethics for nurses and midwives*. London: Nursing and Midwifery Council.

Perry, B (2005) Core nursing values brought to life through stories. *Nursing Standard*, **7**, 41-48.

Saunders, C (2002) *The Philosophy of Hospice*. In Thompson, N (ed) *Loss and Grief*. Basingstoke: Palgrave Macmillan.

Smith, A (2003) Learning about reflection. PhD thesis, University of Northumbria, Newcastle upon Tyne.

Tusaie, K and Dyer, J (2004) Resilience: a historical review of the construct. *Holistic Nursing Practice* **18**, 3-8.

Turnbull James, K (2011). *Leadership in Context: Lessons from new leadership theory and current leadership development practice* [online]. Available at **www.kingsfund.org/leadershipcommission**. (last accessed 27/03/2112).

Watts, D and Morgan, G (1994) Malignant alienation: dangers for patients who are hard to like. *British Journal of Psychiatry*, 164, 11-15.

Watson, J (1988) *Nursing: Human science and human care. A theory of nursing*. New York: National League for Nursing.

Wicks, R (2006) *Overcoming Secondary Stress in Medical and Nursing Practice*. New York: Oxford University Press.

Wilkes, G (2002) Introduction: a second generation of resilience research. *Journal of Clinical Psychology* **58**, 229-232.

Wilkin, K & Slevin, E (2004) The meaning of caring to nurses: an investigation into the nature of caring work in an intensive care unit. *Journal of Clinical Nursing* **13**, 50-59.

Wright, S (2006) Spirited approach. *Nursing Standard* **20**, 24-25.

Chapter 8
The BOND framework of compassionate care

LEARNING OBJECTIVES

By the end of this chapter you should have an understanding of:

1. An overview of the caring indicators that were summarised at the end of previous chapters
2. Aspects of caring, which we have categorised in the themes of: Being and becoming, Overcoming obstacles, Noticing and Doing
3. An initial framework from which you can further develop your understanding of the nature of caring and of ways in which you can enhance your caring skills

Introduction

The indicators highlighted at the end of each chapter, which emerged as a result of our discussions, helped us to focus on the nature of compassionate caring. We brought all the indicators together and then found that we could categorise them into four key themes:-

1. Being and becoming
2. Overcoming obstacles
3. Noticing
4. Doing

Caring is about connecting to others and we found that the initial letters of these four themes reflected this important aspect by forming the apt word BOND (see Figure 8.1 for a diagram of BOND framework below and the appendix for the categorisation of caring indicators under theme headings). In this chapter we have outlined the main characteristics that describe each of the four themes. We hope this framework will assist you in your process of understanding, appreciating and articulating caring with compassion, which is at the heart of effective nursing practice.

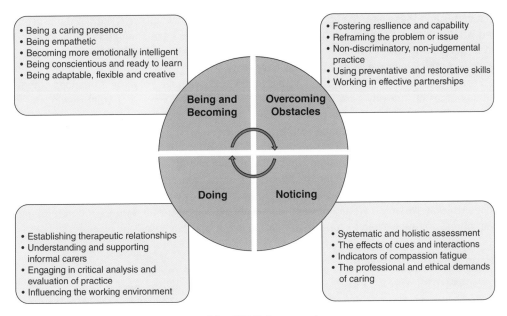

Figure 8.1 Themes and key features of the BOND framework

Looking at the BOND framework

Our aim is to provide you with an initial framework that you can use to develop your under-standing of the nature of compassionate caring and of ways in which you can enhance your caring skills. We hope you will find opportunities to use the framework to discover more about caring throughout your career, as this search for learning should be a never-ending journey. The framework therefore is meant as a prompt for continuation of learning rather than a finished product. The simplicity of the framework is a strength but also a limitation. Another point of consideration is that, although we have categorised the indicators into spe-cific themes, you will find that many overlap as, for example, *who* you *are* influences *how* you *act*. However, this framework is an attempt to simplify the intricacies and sometimes hidden aspects of therapeutic care. You may also find it useful to revisit the detail of the caring indicators and see how we have categorised them within the themes (see Appendix). We are sure you will find more dimensions and characteristics for yourself, if you continue to unravel and analyse the complexity of compassionate caring. For the moment we will look back on our discussions and make our summary of the content within the BOND framework.

Caring by being and becoming

As we have seen throughout the text, caring is linked with what we are like as people. In nursing we learn 'to be and become' (perhaps you've noticed how much you have changed in order to perform your role) as well as learning about the knowledge and practice skills required. Throughout your career you will experience many different situations and challenges and these may lead to reappraisals of how you view yourself, both in the present and what you might become in the future. You may find you are changing in your perceptions, perhaps of others or about what you see as important in your life. Many of your hopes, fears and aspirations are likely to change over time.

From the stories outlined in the chapters in this text, we have seen the influences of individual nurses on the way care is experienced. Our beliefs, values and characteristics affect our identity and how we are perceived as both individuals and professionals. In nursing we attach a great deal of importance to the therapeutic use of 'self' and inherent within this is a recognition of what we bring to situations and interactions with others in a positive sense. However, we have also seen ways in which we can affect others in a negative way. The theme of 'being and becoming' highlights the active search in which we need to engage in order to understand ourselves and develop awareness of what we are and how this influences the way we act. If we understand ourselves we will be better able to understand and help others so that we can ensure we are caring in our approaches.

Being a caring presence

To demonstrate this we have seen that we must be ready to 'connect to' and be 'available for' patients, families and significant others. In doing so, we will be acknowledging our common humanity and ourselves and others as 'spiritual' beings. This means it is possible to see caring as a deep experience that is shared and which some may see as a 'spiritual union'. This is a great privilege for us as nurses and is one that you may be interested in researching further in the future. To us, spirituality in nursing, regardless of whether or not we are religious, includes the opportunities to share with others in their search for meaning and hope. We have found that each caring relationship is a two-way process. The stories also tell us that there is likely to be an exchange of emotional gifts and we need to be aware of and appreciate the benefits gained by us as carers as well as those being cared for. We need therefore to avoid falling into the trap of being professionally arrogant but recognise that as professionals we are part of a continuum of care often in partnership with informal carers.

Being empathetic in order to 'tune into' and help others

Being empathetic means we move our gaze (or focus and concentration) from the body (as an object of intervention) to the person (the individual living a life). The indicators point to the way in which we are able to connect to others through using our communication skills which may include the effective use of touch, humour and silence. It also means being respectful to others, irrespective of their age, gender, cultural origins, class, status or the condition from which they suffer. The stories indicated that the skills of empathy also include being alert to client 'readiness' for information or life changes and listening to their experiences and concerns.

Becoming more emotionally intelligent and competent

We have found that we need to become more aware of and analytical about ourselves - recognising and learning from our own emotions and their effects. Becoming more emotionally intelligent enables us to become more caring by recognising the positive and negative effects of our emotional responses. For example, we can understand the effects of significant incidents in practice such as those relationships in which immediate rapport is established (described as 'clicking') and those in which we make assumptions that lead to non-therapeutic behaviour. We can increase our self-awareness by learning from feelings such as anger, frustration, fears, guilt and sadness. We can manage these emotions and retain balance not by suppressing them, but by learning ways in which we can become more self-controlled, keeping disruptive or overwhelming emotions and impulses in check so that we can carry on with our work of helping others. This is all part of the ethical demands of caring. In doing so, we will increase our competency in coping with situations and therefore increase our self-confidence. We also found that individuals learn from factors that motivate and influence them such as hope and determination and so it is important to become more aware of and acknowledge our capabilities and resources. It is only too easy to dwell on our limitations rather than our strengths.

Being conscientious and ready to learn

As we have seen in the stories, being conscientious often involves going the 'extra mile' and also being ready to take personal responsibility for our caring work. It means that we are prepared to engage in emotional as well as physical labour. By being conscientious, we will also be motivated and committed, compassionate, genuine, warm and sensitive.

The indicators also demonstrate that we have to be open to learning from a wide variety of sources, including patients and their carers, colleagues, professional guidelines, policies and research. The readiness to learn ourselves will also motivate our readiness to help others learn.

Being adaptable, flexible and creative

We are able to become more caring by drawing on personal resources such as our creativity or innovative thinking and by making the most of opportunities to show we care. We can also develop our creativity and imagination in different ways by using a range of resources including perhaps literature, art, poetry and music and by learning to reflect in a number of different ways, including on the lived experience of service users, carers and colleagues.

Caring by overcoming obstacles

We know that the very nature of nursing work means that we meet many problems and obstacles. These may be both personally derived (related to our thoughts, feelings, beliefs and attitudes) and situation derived (perhaps due to pressure and the nature of our workload, organisational constraints and influences, or team conflicts). From the stories that triggered our discussions, we have identified not only a number of obstacles that nurses have to overcome in order to be or remain caring but also a range of strategies that can assist us to do this. Taking problems home may have an adverse impact on our personal relationships and social life; and conversely we may also experience problematic and demanding life events that can impact on the way we act professionally.

Fostering resilience and capability

One of the ways in which we can develop our resilience so that we have more hardiness and ability to cope with workplace adversity and stress is to maintain or gain a positive self-concept. As we have seen, this can influence the ways in which we respond to others and also to challenging situations. We must learn to be aware of and value our strengths, capabilities and available resources. Reflecting on these will enable us to move from problems to solutions and learn ways of developing a range of positive coping strategies so that our self-confidence is enhanced. Another way of caring for ourselves and increasing our overall emotional resilience is utilising other strategies such as maintaining a balance between work and other aspects of our lives, engaging in relaxing and de-stressing activities, taking notice of helpful feedback, and building up 'nurturing' relationships perhaps with peers, mentors or supervisors and other colleagues.

Reframing the problem or issue

We have found that in situations that engender an emotional response within us (e.g. fear, frustration, anger, disappointment, sadness) we are sometimes unable to think or act clearly or rationally. The stress becomes distress and blocks our ability to manage the situation effectively. One of the key ways of changing a distressing situation into a manageable one is to alter how we think about and perceive it, in other words, reframe it. A good example might be changing perceptions that we have of limitations in our knowledge or skills into opportunities for learning. In Chapter 7, we saw how a student was able to use her fears and anxieties about her perceived deficiencies as a useful starting point for her development. With help, she was able to reframe her problems using a solution-focused approach. We also saw how similar approaches helped patients.

We found that when we are caring for others there may be barriers in communication that need to be recognised and overcome. Reframing issues and seeing people as people, not as problems, will be a first step in achieving this. There may also be occasions when we need to suspend our judgement of another's behaviour and lifestyle. We are always in danger of using our various professional or personal frameworks as explanations rather than listening enough to patients and their families. In doing so we may make assumptions and jump to hasty and even inappropriate conclusions. Caring therefore means being closely attentive to others and open-minded enough to consider alternative explanations and approaches – an ongoing process of reframing.

Maintaining non-discriminatory, non-judgemental practice

As we have seen, stereotyping and prejudice can impede effective communication and prevent the establishment of therapeutic relationships. It is therefore an important obstacle to compassionate caring and one that we must recognise in ourselves and in others. There are ways in which we can learn to become more culturally aware and competent but it is important to view every individual as a unique blend of values, beliefs, attitudes, history and culture. The NMC Code (2008) reinforces this by indicating that 'you must not discriminate in any way against those in your care and that you must demonstrate a personal and professional commitment to equality and diversity'. Our stories have also taught us a great deal about the effects of unequal power and vulnerability. It would seem that listening to what people say is a compelling and informative way of forming a firm basis for compassionate, individualised care.

Using preventative and restorative skills

Proactive interventions and risk assessments are an essential part of the preventative caring process. However, in the rush and bustle of routines and procedures something obvious can easily be missed or assumptions can be made. With a focus on completing tasks in a limited amount of time, the 'person' may be lost and important opportunities for the nurturing and restorative/healing aspects of nursing care missed. As we found in Chapter 4, it may be quiet and compliant patients who may not gain the care they need because they were not asked. Not only does proactive care engender trust and feelings of being safe and cared for, but it also helps prevent problems occurring in the first place. Using strategies such as intentional rounding may be a useful monitoring tool for this.

As we have seen, we may also 'lose' the person because of the way we perceive them as problems, particularly if they are hostile and aggressive. We can be helped by policies and organisational procedures such as those related to 'zero tolerance' and handling difficult situations. Perspectives and guidance can also be gained from academic knowledge and also through undertaking shared reflective activities. This will widen our understanding and increase our skills in preventing and managing such challenges. We know from our discussions how important it is for any individual to feel cared for even if they show behaviour that is challenging or problematic for us. If anyone does not feel cared for, this can have a negative impact on his or her self-image and their ability to cope with illness, anxieties or adversity. In working with patients and their families, we need to understand that there are times of particular stress that may occur, perhaps during life transitions or periods of frustration, loss and change. The indicators stress the importance of communicating sensitively and effectively, listening to and exchanging information and knowledge with patients and carers, overcoming any barriers so they can make their feelings and needs known. We can work in partnership with patients, relatives and colleagues to help them find and use their strengths and resources to overcome difficulties or adjust to new challenges.

Working in effective partnerships

We have to overcome obstacles to our ability to be caring, which may sometimes be related to organisational pressures and demands from wider socio-political and economic factors. Because of the inevitably rapidly changing world of health and social care, it is important that individual members of health and social care teams value each other and the particular contribution each can make. We need to find ways of articulating to others the importance of the caring work we as nurses undertake so that it achieves the recognition it deserves. However, we can accomplish only so much on our own. For example, we have included a number of stories about the care of older people where the role of nurses in delivering direct care is critical, but positive outcomes also depend on nurses working effectively with the older person, his or her family and the multidisciplinary/multi-agency team. We can overcome obstacles and achieve much more if we are members of cohesive and collaborative teams, working in partnership with patients and their families. We need all the knowledge and skills of the teams and relatives and carers so they can be used for the good of the patient or client. Working together and gaining trust and respect for team members, discussing problems openly and honestly will help develop effective teamwork, overcome obstacles to seamless care and enhance the patient experience.

Caring by noticing

The caring indicators have shown us the importance of 'noticing' - picking up cues that may be otherwise hidden. This sensitivity to others is at the centre of our ability to communicate effectively and show empathy and compassion. We have to use our senses (sight, hearing, smell and touch) to notice, and also our interpretations and feelings about people and situations, which may be almost 'unconscious' (or intuitive). However, at times we may not 'notice', perhaps deliberately as a defence mechanism, to prevent us from getting involved or because we are focusing on tasks that have to be achieved in a very short time.

We can use a variety of reflective activities in order to learn more about the art of noticing. In doing so, we can increase our sensitivity and awareness. We will widen and enhance our caring skills if we also use our observation skills to notice and learn from the ways in which others undertake effective caring interventions, such as our professional colleagues or informal carers.

Noticing as part of systematic and holistic assessment and decision making

Noticing is a key skill in nursing, particularly in systematic and holistic assessment. Nurses need to engage in complex observations and interactions continuously. They need to be particularly sensitive if they are to be able to pick up not only the obvious, but also the more subtle or hidden, cues, which may be physical, emotional, spiritual, educational or social in origin. The stories have also indicated that effective nurses are able to notice when there are opportunities for establishing connectedness in relationships with patients and others. For example, they use skills in being able to recognise when a client and their family are in a state of 'readiness' for supportive help, information and health education. They are also sensitive to religious and cultural needs and preferences and are proactive by asking patients what they need. In addition, they make every effort to notice the effects of their interactions in order to develop optimum emotional and physical health in others.

Noticing the effects of cues and interactions

We have learned that some interactions trigger certain responses within us and we can learn a great deal from these. In Chapter 4, for example, we found that identification with particular patients and objects can act as triggers and affect our emotional balance. We may be reminded of someone close to us or of some other aspect of our own life. Noticing and articulating these feelings may help us to care for ourselves and avoid compassion fatigue or distancing ourselves and becoming 'hard'. In doing so, we will be better able to remain caring in our approach to others.

As we discussed earlier, we found that with some patients we may establish an immediate rapport. This may be beneficial in that it helps us to interact with a degree of ease, but it can be problematic if we fail to notice that we may be moving outside the parameters of our professional relationship. We need to notice how we are reacting to situations or to others and learn from both our positive and negative emotions. There are examples throughout the text of students and nurses who have learned a great deal from their negative but common emotions of guilt, dislike, anger and perhaps even disgust. We must recognise that we all have such feelings and thoughts at times and must accept that we have a 'shadow side'. Nurses are not miracle workers or angels and the stories have helped us to understand that we need to learn to be able to cope with disappointment or any other negative feelings we might have. In addition, we have found that what we think we might be like in the future (our 'possible selves') can be not only motivational but also based on hidden and sometimes irrational fears.

Noticing is an integral part of self-awareness, essential if we are to make rational judgements of our capabilities and reactions. We have suggested that we need to apply the same kind of critical analysis to ourselves as that which we use in our academic work. Indeed, the 'art of noticing' has been described by Boud and Walker (1990) as a principal component of reflection.

We have also found many examples of the importance service users place on feeling that they were noticed. Van der Cingel (2011) found this in her research, in which she explored the notion of compassion in care with older adults. She found they mentioned 'attentiveness' most often as an indicator of this. She discussed how the patients 'noticed' when a nurse was 'noticing' them,

> *'The first thing that comes to mind in thinking about compassion concerns approaching the other person as a human being. Such a contact immediately compels a nurse to act, however small or non-verbal this act may be. Acts such as making eye contact, or slowing your pace, or pulling up a chair to sit next to the bed, are an invitation to the patient. This shows that there is a conscious wish for contact; the nurse gives her "permission" to continue.' (page 676)*

It would therefore seem that showing that we are focused on patients and paying them attention is one of the most important aspects of caring in that it is from this that trust and many other indicators of compassionate caring begin.

Noticing indicators of compassion fatigue

Nurses experience all kinds of demanding situations and pressures that can lead to excessive stress. This is an important issue for quality care, as research by Rafferty *et al.* (2007) has shown. The best-staffed UK NHS Trusts had significantly lower patient mortality rates than the least-well-staffed Trusts. It was also found that on better-staffed wards, employees had significantly lower levels of 'burn-out' and higher levels of job satisfaction. Other research has reinforced this. For example, Najjarn *et al.* (2009) showed that compassion fatigue takes a toll, not only on the health care provider, but also on the workplace, causing decreased productivity, more sick days and higher turnover of staff.

We have highlighted the importance of recognising and managing stress and of looking after ourselves by developing the ability to 'bounce back' when meeting challenges or adversity (see Chapter 7). It is also vital to notice the effects of particularly stressful periods on colleagues and we need to pay attention to emotional and behavioural cues that may indicate this. If we think that care is being adversely affected as a result, we must communicate this to appropriate others and seek help so action can be taken. As a member of a multi-professional team, noticing indicators of stress is an important way of caring for each other. As we found in Chapter 5, it is also important to notice indicators of compassion fatigue in informal carers and find ways of helping them to maintain the positive benefits of providing care.

Noticing the professional and ethical demands of caring

We began collecting stories because of our own, and students' and colleagues', concerns about incidents in which they felt their ability to provide quality care was sometimes compromised. Both nurses and service users gave us stories of incidents that had occurred a number of years ago, which they had not discussed with anyone but still thought about. Once these incidents were analysed, they found there may have been unrealistic expectations of themselves, or they recognised that more could have been achieved or undertaken in a different manner. These incidents were often not dramatic events but everyday happenings.

Ethical debates and professional concerns were there but needed to be reflected upon, analysed and in some cases acted upon.

Many of the stories we used in this text also raised a number of ethical considerations and we found that a variety of resources, including the NMC Code of Professional Conduct, helped to guide us in our discussions about professional behaviour. There are professional and ethical demands on nurses not to ignore but to notice areas of concern and respond in an appropriate professional manner. This may mean voicing concerns through appropriate channels, for example about overwhelming pressures, inadequate resources or training. If necessary it may lead to 'whistle-blowing' in an informed and considered way. All of this takes a certain amount of courage, energy and ability to negotiate assertively. The *Front Line Care Report* (2010:28) highlighted the importance of nurses developing these skills: 'Nurses and midwives told us they were still often regarded as passive implementers of others' policies, and had to fight many times over for their place at the top table. High quality care for all will not be achieved unless policy-makers, leaders, managers, and nurses and midwives themselves change this mindset and become active, equal partners and change agents.'

Caring by doing

This is the aspect that demonstrates to others our skills in caring. All aspects of the framework are interrelated (or are bonded) to each other and help reveal what caring is really all about. Nurses must undertake various tasks and activities with a high level of practical expertise and skill; but without the scientific knowledge and artistry required for holistic care for the person (illuminated by the caring indicators) such nursing actions may fall short of what service users need and expect. Caring relationships are founded on good, safe practice. This means engaging in reflective, lifelong learning and ongoing professional development to ensure the provision of effective, skilful, safe and compassionate care.

Preparing the ground for and maintaining therapeutic relationships

Trust is an essential requirement for a caring, therapeutic relationship. As we have seen from the stories, in nursing this may have to be established within a very short period of time. This does not necessarily mean that the relationship between nurse and patient has to be at a very deep level, although, as we have learned, on many occasions interactions can become very meaningful. This is in line with Bassett (2002), who concludes that special 'bonds' may or may not occur between nurse and patient and that although closeness brings with it mutual benefits, without it 'good' nursing care can still be given. However, we have found evidence that caring behaviours are important from the very start of interactions with patients and their relatives (whether they become 'deep' or remain at a 'superficial' level). Our indicators confirmed there are benefits to be gained from participating in informal social exchange and in simple acts of kindness that show others we are interested in and value them. We can develop trust and provide reassurance by being available and giving other people confidence both in our technical skills and in our ability to listen to and help them. We have seen the importance of responding to the concerns and distress of patients and their families and helping to reduce their pain, whether it is physical, emotional or spiritual.

Indicators also highlight the importance of interventions that help each service user to develop and retain a sense of personal worth, and feelings of acceptability and hope. We must promote and maintain caring relationships by engaging in anti-discriminatory practice and in doing so help others to maintain their self-respect and dignity. We have found that caring can be a spiritual union in which deep experience is shared and that we can help others in their search for comfort, meaning and hope. Respecting their religious beliefs, facilitating the meeting of their needs and practices are all part of the caring process.

Much can be achieved through engaging in skilled verbal and non-verbal communication, responding and attending to detail in a 'care-ful' way. It is of particular importance to listen to how people describe their situation and lived experience. In this way we 'tune in' to them and use and develop our skills of empathy. The stories give us a great deal of information about how nurses can turn their compassion into effective nursing actions, for example the ways in which they help to change distressing situations into more manageable ones. This may include helping others to adapt and cope with change and to function at their optimal level.

Understanding and supporting informal carers

The importance of entering into equitable and non-patronising partnerships with informal carers has been highlighted in many of the stories. In order for effective multi-professional, multi-agency care to succeed, patients and carers need to be of central importance. There are often competing demands on carers and we found that professionals must engage in activities that take into account the whole 'family' and provide emotional support for them as required, particularly if they have to adapt and cope with change. Working in partnership with informal carers means valuing and using their knowledge and skills. It could also involve teaching and supporting them so that they can achieve quite complex practical skills and helping them to know how to access and negotiate for other resources. In this way people who are providing significant care can be helped to gain and share knowledge and 'power'. They are then more likely to retain the benefits of caring and continue to provide this essential part of the care continuum.

Critical evaluation and analysis of practice

Throughout the previous chapters we have made the point that a caring nurse engages in critical and analytical reflection. In this way nurses gain knowledge for and from practice. We have seen the importance of creating an open and caring environment for service users, carers and also staff to provide a culture of compassionate care. This can be developed through excellent role modelling, and the passing on of tacit practice knowledge. Tacit knowledge is particularly important as practice changes and less direct care is undertaken by qualified nurses, but they retain the responsibility for guiding, supporting and monitoring staff and evaluating the quality of care they provide.

It is through examination and analysis that we find new ways of 'seeing' and 'doing', vital for evaluating whether care is effective and compassionate. Reflection can be part of this process and helps us uncover aspects of caring that might otherwise be hidden. For example, as we saw in Charlie and Bella's story in Chapter 4, effective communication was achieved by engaging in a 'dance of rhythmic harmony'. Critical analysis of this practice situation using academic perspectives helped with our understanding. Reflecting on and sharing stories such as this help to uncover and pass on tacit or hidden practice knowledge, articulating and adding to our caring skills. This knowledge can be passed on to others as well as uncovering our capabilities and areas for further development. Throughout the text we have described various techniques and strategies we can use for professional growth including dialogue with and support from mentors and clinical supervisors, peer support, group discussion, reflective journals and the use of imagery and metaphor.

Influencing the working environment

We have noted that in order to care for others we have to be nurtured ourselves. As we have seen, individual reflection with the help of a 'critical' friend or colleagues will help us to gain self-understanding and the confidence to overcome our fears, misconceptions and misgivings. The support we gain from our peers, family and friends should not be underestimated so we need to make time for them and for wider pursuits that help us to maintain equilibrium through achieving a healthy work-life balance. If we neglect these important aspects of our lives we will not be able to care effectively or influence a working environment that is conducive to compassionate care.

Over one hundred years ago, Florence Nightingale considered that the most important aspect of nursing was to create the conditions under which a person could be healed by nature or by God (Nightingale, 1969). An environment can be healing if we care 'with' as well as care 'for' a patient and their family. Then we are, as Barker and Buchanan-Barker (2004) suggest, helping individuals to grow and develop by giving them literal and metaphorical 'nourishment' which lies at the root of nursing. To do this we need to draw on both the scientific and the artistic knowledge base for nursing. Service users need to feel safe and are entitled to skilled, evidence-based interventions, including the prompt meeting of fundamental needs such as hygiene, nutrition and pain relief. A caring nurse therefore needs to keep up to date, be highly skilled in technical procedures and be able to understand, engage in, utilise and evaluate the relevance of research findings. The caring indicators have highlighted the importance of the art of nursing, since that is the aspect of caring that is so easily taken for granted or not understood. As we have seen, however, this is not an indulgence but an imperative and should have equal weighting with the science of nursing. Expertise in technical skills without attending to the person can be detrimental to the healing process, just as would 'sympathy' without a knowledgeable skills base.

The practice setting can influence the way we care for and with others. If the atmosphere is one of distrust, disorganisation and lacks warmth and collegiality, it will be stressful for both the cared-for as well as for those providing the care. Everyone can make a contribution to this influential environment – not only by the way in which each contributes to care but also by the ways in which they support and work with colleagues, keep 'cool' in stressful situations, use humour appropriately and assist in developing others as well as themselves.

Using the BOND framework

We have included the following scenario, which occurred when we were undertaking a group tutorial with a number of nursing students after they had completed a practice placement. We used the BOND framework to help them analyse the situation.

Case Study 8.1

The students commented that they felt they were 'drowning' in the heavy workload and were feeling emotionally drained and worn out. They said they were glad to be back in the university as it gave them a break from the emotional and physical demands of placement. They started talking about guilt feelings, saying they believed they had sometimes not responded enough to patient needs. They also shared examples of how they had been affected emotionally, for example when caring for dying and very ill patients and also when they had to help distressed relatives and, in empathising with them, identified with their experiences. After becoming upset following a particularly harrowing episode, Paula, one of the students, commented that she had been told by a staff nurse that 'nurses have to be hard' and that she was 'too soft and too caring'.

To think about

+ Consider the incident described above. What aspects do Paula and the other students need to think about in order to understand how being caring has consequences for the nurse in terms of emotional stability and how can nurses manage this? Do they need to be hard to survive?
+ You might want to use parts of the BOND framework to help with your reflections and also you might want to draw on pertinent literature to help with a deeper analysis.

Compare your considerations with those of our students

We found the BOND framework gave us pointers to help in our reflective discussion with the students. When Paula first said that she had been told that 'nurses have to be hard', a number of the other students agreed with this to some extent. We asked them to look at the BOND framework and consider the 'being and becoming' theme. All agreed that they wanted to continue to be a caring presence, and be able to show they were empathetic as outlined in the caring indicators. They recognised the importance of developing these and overcoming the 'being hard' obstacles by finding effective ways of managing their emotions. However, they had also noticed ('noticing' is the third theme of the framework) that they had become emotionally and physically drained and recognised that this could lead to compassion fatigue. They suggested that they could use these feelings as an incentive for understanding better why this had occurred. They recognised that it was important to move on to the final theme of the framework of doing something positive to manage their feelings. Considering the 'caring by doing' theme helped them to see that they had not been caring for themselves adequately, for example by having too high expectations of themselves and also having unrealistic feelings that they had to make everyone feel better.

One student commented that the framework themes were all interrelated in that you needed to notice what you were doing, be conscientious about uncovering and 'dealing with obstacles' (the second theme), be a caring person to yourself as well as for others in order to be what you wanted to be. We all thought this comment, although rather convoluted, helped us understand some of the complexity and 'work' needed in order to be and become a caring nurse.

We used the opportunity to help the students to go on further with their critical analysis by using imagery and metaphor to think again about what it meant to be 'hard'. They decided that something that is hard, although it might be tough, could also be inflexible and brittle and so would be likely to break under pressure. They thought that people who were hard were often insensitive, unkind, forceful, and sometimes self-centred and ruthless. Some nurses appeared 'hard' when they distanced themselves from others and became task-oriented rather than person-centred, probably to avoid feeling vulnerable and getting hurt. The students said they hoped that they wouldn't be like that even when they had more responsibilities in the future. They discussed whether this hardness might be a sign of 'professional burn-out' and possibly could be the end result of being too 'soft' and overwhelmed with emotions. This process would have an adverse effect on the individual nurse and would also affect their ability to help patients, relatives and colleagues as much as they should. One student commented that she had read somewhere that nurses have to have a degree of 'hardiness' rather than being hard. The other students liked this description as it helped them to reframe the issue, conjuring up a different image – one in which the nurse could still be emotionally and therapeutically connected but tough enough to acknowledge his or her limitations and be able to 'bounce back' when feeling under pressure and overwhelmed.

They concluded that the framework itself had helped them to understand that in order to stay caring they could use their emotional responses, understand them and learn different ways of managing them. We advised them to look for academic literature in order to understand more about the nature of emotional intelligence, particularly in its relationship with personal resilience. We provided them with Tusaie and Dyer's (2004:3) definition of emotional resilience (see Chapter 7): 'a combination of abilities and characteristics that interact dynamically and allow an individual to bounce back, cope successfully and function above the norm in spite of significant stress or adversity'. We also discussed work by Abraham (2004), who indicated that memory functions best when the mind is calm, influencing our capacity to pay attention and pick up cues.

The students commented that they could more easily look back calmly and critically reflect when they were away from the situation. Although they acknowledged that reflection is part of good practice, in the rush and bustle of everyday working life it is often easier to reflect more systematically and get things into 'better proportion' when away from the situation. One student suggested that keeping a personal diary helped her to do this.

Time to think back

Did you find you could relate to the experiences of our students? You may have found your considerations took you down a similar path to ours, but don't worry if you took a different stance. You may have extended your knowledge by undertaking a literature search, perhaps by using key words such as 'stress/stress management', 'emotional intelligence', 'hardiness', 'emotional resilience', 'emotional labour', 'burn-out'.

Summary

In this chapter we have provided an overview of the caring indicators summarised at the end of each chapter. These were derived from stories told to us by patients and their relatives, students and qualified nurses. We found there were numerous indicators that often confirmed research findings and perspectives from academic literature but were brought to life and reassessed for their relevance to caring in practice. We found that categorising them into four main themes helped to clarify and encapsulate what a caring nurse is and does. These were:

1. Being and becoming
2. Overcoming obstacles
3. Noticing
4. Doing

The initial BOND framework for caring could be used to develop your understanding further. Remember that frameworks are there just to help us; they are not complete answers but can be useful tools for developing our understanding and behaviour. Although the aspects of caring we have outlined are applicable to many situations and contexts in which nurses presently work, the world of practice continues to change dramatically. Our caring skills need to evolve to meet the challenge of these changes and that is why it is so important to ensure that analytical and reflective caring discourse continues.

Looking forward

In Chapter 9, we will review the journey of learning we have made throughout this text and consider the importance of continuing to maintain compassionate caring as a key aspect of nursing, whatever the future holds for the profession.

Activity

Look for caring moments in practice and consider one of these, for example an interaction between a nurse and a patient or carer. Try using the BOND framework to help with your reflections and draw on relevant literature which will help you achieve a deeper analysis.

References

Abraham, R (2004) Emotional competence as antecedent to performance: a contingency framework. *Genetic, Social and General Psychology Monographs* **130**, 117–143.

Barker, P and Buchanan-Barker, P (2004) Caring as a craft. *Nursing Standard* **19**, 17–18.

Bassett, C (2002) Nurses' perceptions of care and caring. *International Journal of Nursing Practice* **8**, 8-15.

Boud, D and Walker, D (1990) Making the most of experience. *Studies in Continuing Education* **12**, 61-80.

http://webarchive.nationalarchives.gov.uk/20100331110400/http:/cnm.independent.gov.uk/ (last accessed 4/06/2012).

Najjar, N, Davis, L, Beck-Coon K, Carney Doebbeling, C (2009) Compassion Fatigue: a review of the research to date and relevance to cancer -care providers. Journal of Health Psychology **14**, 267-277 .

Nightingale, F (1969) *Notes on Nursing: what it is and what it is not.* New York: Dover. (First published in 1860.)

NMC (Nursing and Midwifery Council) (2008) The Code: Standards of conduct, performance and ethics for nurses and midwives. London: Nursing and Midwifery Council.

Rafferty, A, Clarke, S, Coles, J, Ball, J, James, P, McKee, M, Aiken, L (2007) Outcomes of variation in hospital nurse staffing in English hospitals: cross-sectional analysis of survey data and discharge records. *International Journal of Nursing Studies* **44** (2): 175-82.

Tusaie, K and Dyer, J (2004) Resilience: a historical review of the construct. *Holistic Nursing Practice* **18**, 3-8.

Van der Cingel, M (2011) Compassion in care: A qualitative study of older people with a chronic disease and nurses *Nursing Ethics* **18** (5): 672-685

Chapter 9
Looking back and moving forward

LEARNING OBJECTIVES

The purpose of this chapter is to review:

1. The importance of stories within the discourse of compassionate caring

2. A framework for creating and maintaining a culture of compassionate caring

3. The importance of ensuring that nursing knowledge and compassionate practice are developed within organisational changes and shifting professional boundaries

4. Nursing work in terms of emotional and social capital

Introduction

In this final chapter we will review our journey and consider again what we have learned about the nature of caring and the part stories from patients, carers and colleagues can play in our reflective analysis and evaluation of that care. The powerful effect of stories is evident in some of the media coverage concerning shortcomings in care but they are also an important resource for research, although we need to remind ourselves about the hazards and pitfalls of storytelling. We need to face issues related to the capacity for nurses to continue to care with compassion so that this is not lost within future organisational changes and shifting professional boundaries. According to *Front Line Care* (Department of Health 2010:3) 'A carequake is fast approaching: the massive and growing requirement to provide skilled care for people with many different needs – arising from long-term conditions, drug and alcohol addiction, the complex needs of ageing, problems in the early years, and much more. Nurses are centre stage to meet these needs and must be properly equipped and supported to do so.'

Reviewing our journey

In this text, we have journeyed together and begun to unravel some of the many dimensions of caring which we see as encompassing both the art and the science of nursing. Writing this textbook has reinforced for us that the artistry of nursing is highly important and must be integrated into the application of scientific knowledge and technical skills. This is the only way we can provide compassionate care. Scientific and technical knowledge and the ability to engage in complex skills are exciting and have high status but the art of compassionate caring may be taken for granted, not well articulated and its significance overlooked. We hope you have found that the stories have led you to appreciate once more that sometimes, even every day, fundamental tasks create important opportunities for caring, which can be as engaging and therapeutic as undertaking complex interventions. It is in these very 'basic' tasks that nursing as a profession has been found wanting, in spite of many examples of excellent practice and compassionate care. The concern is to find ways of ensuring that we not only recognise the indicators of compassionate care but that we engage with and guide others to whom we delegate care.

We have found that stories have been central to our ability to uncover the art of nursing. Tschudin (1999:198) defines an artist as not only one who paints, sculpts or is a creative cook but anyone who undertakes 'any gesture or act that takes us beyond ourselves and opens our physical and inner eyes to something more than the obvious'. The stories from service users, carers, students and qualified nursing staff have done just this – enabling us to see things in a new light – and have generated understandings of aspects that might otherwise have been hidden from our view.

Our thoughts about the importance of stories

We have used stories from service users throughout this text. In their Point of Care review paper, Goodrich and Cornwell (2008:7) describe the importance of this within a society in which information is more readily shared:-

> 'Patients' stories bring the experience to life and make it accessible to other people. The growth of social networking websites, along with the contemporary appetite for publicising personal experiences that previously would have been considered too private or too intimate to share, makes it likely this will continue.'

We know that stories have had a strong influence on changing public perceptions of nurses and other health-care professionals. We have to accept their influence and try to use them to see what problems and issues they are reflecting, or perhaps how and why misconceptions might have arisen. This information provides the impetus and pointers for improvement of practice and service delivery.

As in everyday life, stories have an important influence on the way in which we and others perceive and therefore construct nursing. From the very beginning of the text, we learned about the value of stories as rich learning experiences in our professional life and through them we began our journey into a discourse about compassionate caring. From the stories we were able to identify significant caring moments that occurred in busy traumatic periods but also in everyday situations.

To think about

Stories are very powerful and very useful but there are some hazards and pitfalls associated with them.

✦ What do you think they are? Make particular reference to your professional life and make a few notes. If you get stuck you may find Chapter 1 helpful.

Compare your considerations with ours

We hope you will find similarities but don't worry if you have come to some different conclusions. Stories are told for a purpose. The way we tell and reflect on our stories depends on who is listening to us. An easy way of considering this is to use the key words of what, when, why, where, how and who. As we noted in Chapter 1, stories are socially reconstructed and reflect the content and the expected audience (Mishler, 1991). The stories you use for your reflections as part of an educational course or in clinical supervision are likely to take on a different form from 'storytelling' occurring with a colleague in an informal setting. We think that although using stories to describe your practice experience is useful as part of an academic exercise – in that you can learn valuable lessons from integrating theory and practice and thinking again about your performance – there is a pitfall in that you may be constrained by academic marking criteria and so feel unable to disclose or address particular strong emotional feelings that you have. You may therefore submit a 'sanitised' account. You may have overcome this by finding that you gain most help from sharing your powerful personal stories with your peers or a trusted colleague.

The power of stories can be a disadvantage as well as an advantage. Horror stories or biased views about people and situations can engender fear and distrust. They may form the basis of professional gossip and of unfortunate categorisations such as the 'unpopular' patient, relative, nurse or colleague. For example, perceptions of particular student placements may be based on one particularly scary story or a myth. However, as we have seen in this text, it is helpful to become sensitive and to be honest about what might be our tendency to exaggerate or emphasise (to make the story more interesting or to get sympathy). We will then be able to uncover prejudices or biases that might affect our relationships and behaviour.

We can also get stuck within the emotional content of stories and therefore not use them as effectively as we might if we do not reflect on them at a deeper analytical level. To do this we need to look for a wide variety of perspectives and different forms of evidence. We (as authors) recognised this when we began to consider writing this text about caring in nursing. We knew that any attempt at a simple definition would be inadequate and that the stories would evoke a variety of emotions associated with caring (and indeed uncaring) behaviour. These could be more effectively examined through the use of a wide variety of resources and our examination included theoretical perspectives. We hope that, like us, you have found how interesting and informative this can be.

Stepping into the future

To think about

+ Identify and list changes that you think are likely to occur over the next few years and that could have an impact on the way in which compassionate nursing care can be provided.
+ Pause for a moment to think and then compare your thoughts with the discussion that follows.

It is difficult to predict as the world changes continuously: economically, politically, socially and environmentally. However, our list includes the likelihood of a number of issues.

Funding issues for health and social care will continue and there will remain a focus on value for money and proven effectiveness. The NHS five-year plan (DoH, 2009) identified six challenges faced by all modern health-care systems: ever higher patient expectations; an ageing society; the information age; the changing nature of disease; advances in treatments; and a changing workforce.

Most people will continue to expect to be more involved in their health care and have their ideas and concerns addressed, to be informed about their condition and briefed about treatment risks and benefits (The Health Foundation, 2011). They will expect to be involved in any decisions made about their care and educated and supported in self-care. The *Front Line Care Report* (Department of Health, 2010:28) relates this to a rise in consumerism and a focus on entitlement that 'have raised expectations to a level that would not be recognized by earlier generations. Service users and carers are much more knowledgeable about their conditions, and many want to be more involved in care planning and decision-making.' There are also challenges related to longer life expectancy, increases in birth rate, socio-economic factors, and transient populations.

There will continue to be an emphasis on primary and community health related to pre-ventative interventions to promote health, for example in reducing the number of people who are obese or have alcohol or drug dependency. There is now more emphasis on path-ways of care and patient journeys that cut across primary and secondary care, requiring nurses to negotiate, plan and work with other professions and agencies. There will continue to be more care provided closer to home and within the home environment.

All of these changes provide opportunities to give compassionate care. However, there are also challenges in that to do so caring nurses must be flexible, open to new learning, creative and resilient. They must demonstrate that they can use knowledge, skills and atti-tudes that promote effective partnerships with patients, carers and colleagues. These will involve using interpersonal and communication skills such as listening, negotiating, facili-tating, information–giving, motivating and reassuring – particularly relevant for working with 'people with experience' of long-term conditions. These partnerships, which will often involve multi-professional, multi-agency input, must be based on mutual trust and power sharing.

Other changes are related to increases in technology and scientific and medical knowledge which have resulted in ongoing pressures for more specialisation and advancement of skills for all health-care workers. It is important that there is a willingness to share knowledge and information for the benefit of the patient. For example, there are opportunities with the growth and influence of the internet and electronic tools and devices including those to facilitate record keeping and decision making. In addition, changes in role boundaries, for example through delegation of tasks previously performed by medical staff, related to the changes in technology, will continue to lead to new responsibilities and the required acquisition of new skills for nurses.

The Nursing and Care Quality Forum (2012) suggests that technology needs to free up more time to care and avoid patients being asked the same questions repetitively. Such technology may provide effective and integrated electronic patient records for seamless care through patient journeys. Foster and Hawkins (2005) discuss the effect of the expansion in interactive devices such as clipboards, smart cards, virtual reality, web technology and mobile phone applications. If all these are to be used for the good of the patient, these authors suggest that nurses should not wait for change to occur but should exercise their nursing power and influence decisions about what is needed. They go on to warn that if not, the changes could mean that nurses would spend more time monitoring the collection of data rather than engaging with the physical and emotional care of the patient. If nurses can help direct the development and use of technology to free up nursing time to spend with patients and their families, this will be hugely beneficial. A particular challenge for the nurse will be not only to be able to demonstrate technical knowledge but also use the art of compassionate caring, to engage with each patient so that the person is not lost within all the technology – what we have described earlier as maintaining the 'I-Thou' relationship.

Longley et al. (2007) stressed the importance of working within and across patient pathways and of effective multidisciplinary teams working and reflecting these changes in nursing career pathways. They outlined the possibility of several key opportunities for nurses, including directing and leading care, both within and outside the NHS, using entrepreneurial skills, and asserted that nurses could be at the forefront of initiatives in public health and preventative medicine. To do all this they suggest that 'Nurses will be required to have a high level of knowledge, critical thinking, and autonomy at registration' (Longley et al., 2007:34). Debates about future roles and responsibilities will continue and we need to engage with them if nurses are to influence the future of nursing.

Our work has shown us that service users expect that nurses and others who provide care are caring individuals and this is the key reason most of us would give for coming into nursing. In the future, we must ensure that we do not lose our caring knowledge and skills with any expansion of nursing roles and changes in care provision so that we are able to keep compassionate caring as a central component. We must therefore continue to develop and demonstrate caring behaviours and provide evidence about what difference caring makes to a variety of outcomes including patient experiences and rate of recovery, meeting government and organisational targets and in evaluating quality of care. In the future it would seem that even more direct care may be provided by health-care assistants (or their equivalent). An important part of a nurse leadership role in the future (and one we believe must not be forgotten within a business-orientated, evidence-based health-care system with its myriad pressures and preoccupations) will be to share with them the knowledge and skills nurses have about the art of caring. In this way compassionate caring will survive and grow.

Helping to create and maintain a culture of compassionate care

> ## To think about
>
> Qualified nurses are increasingly expected to develop effective leadership, management and entrepreneurial skills.
>
> + As a leader, what would be the most important factors to consider in order to create and maintain a culture of compassionate care?
> + Pause for a moment to think and then compare your thoughts with the discussion that follows.

You may have come across work by the National Nursing Research Unit, undertaken by Maben with Griffiths (2008), who describe three key aspects of the nurse's role as practitioner, partner, leader, which they see as rooted in the core values and ethos that underpin the profession. Nurses of the future will be:-

+ 'skilled and respected **practitioners** providing effective high quality healthcare across a range of settings;
+ vital and valued **partners** in the delivery of health care – partners in the multidisciplinary team, co-ordinating different resources and skill sets to ensure high quality care, partners with patients and carers in delivering personalised care, and responsible members of the broader healthcare system taking personal responsibility for efficient and effective functioning;
+ confident and effective **leaders** and champions of care quality with a powerful voice at all levels of the healthcare system, from policymaking to the frontline' (Maben with Griffiths 2008:15).

We need, however, to make sure that there is a culture of compassionate care in which nurses fulfil the roles described by Maben and, based on the care indicators within the BOND framework, we have set out what we see as key components for achieving this (see Figure 9.1).

Effective leadership and management

The importance of high-quality management and leadership has been highlighted in the report by the King's Fund Commission (2011). This report defines leadership as the art of motivating a group of people to achieve a common goal and, if we accept this definition, we can see that nurses are required to develop and use leadership skills in many aspects of their work and at many levels of seniority. The report goes on to explain the importance of this. 'Leadership development must not focus purely on technical competencies, but on the ability to create climates in which individuals can themselves act to improve services and care' (King's Fund Commission, 2011:21).

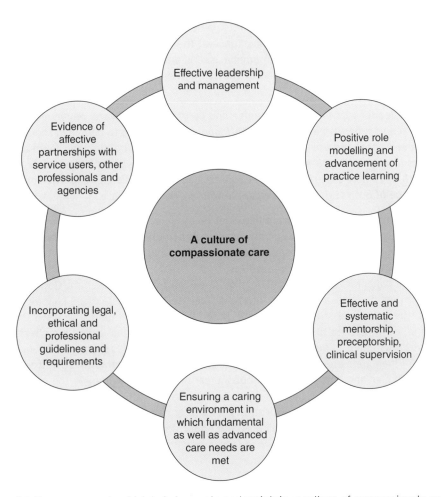

Figure 9.1 Key components which help to create and maintain a culture of compassionate care

All this is in line with the notion of 'distributed leadership' which we introduced (in Chapter 7) and that has been identified as a collective approach of shared responsibility throughout an organisation in contrast to 'top-down', hierarchical, or 'heroic' approaches. More 'fluid' definitions of leadership mean that there are likely to be increases in the recognition or development of various kinds of expertise and skills within an organisation, improving over-all leadership capacity. This approach is important at a time of change in the ways in which health care is commissioned and provided and one in which nurses need to engage, negoti-ate and participate in decision making across a variety of organisations and systems of care. Brigham *et al.* (2012:27) reiterate this, seeing this approach to leadership as 'more conducive to organisational change particularly in the context of emerging ways of working that are based on collaboration, networking and multi-agency working rather than single organisa-tion work'.

Ward leaders and/or managers operating within this context need to be able to create and maintain positive practice environments providing opportunities for development and support for others. If all team members feel valued and cared for, they are more likely to value and care for others. The vital importance of the ward or unit manager or team leader as a linchpin and role model has been emphasised in various reports (Department of Health 2010, 2012) and there are many calls for the strengthening of this role. The report for the Nursing and Care Quality Forum (Department of Health, 2012:4) explains why this is so:-

> 'Having a leader who is able to organise and co-ordinate the ward, department or com-munity team; supervise and support staff; spend time talking to people in their care and their loved ones; and ensure standards are maintained, will build good team dynamics and result in positive care outcomes. A visible leader who has managerial experience, a wealth of clinical experience and is able to lead by example can gain the respect and confidence of both staff and those people who are receiving care.'

However, important though the ward manager or team leader is in helping to create a cul-ture of caring and acting as a role model, as we noted in Chapter 7, ensuring high standards of compassionate care is the responsibility of each individual within a care team and the management of the organisation as a whole.

In a review paper for the King's Fund Point of Care Programme, Goodrich and Cornwell (2008) argued that action is needed at four different levels to create sustainable change in health services: the individual staff member; the team, unit or department; the institution as a whole and the wider health-care system. Senior leaders, including board members, senior executives and senior clinicians shape the culture of the organisation by influencing 'the priorities of managers and staff, how they behave towards each other and towards patients and their families and how staff feel about the services they provide and the organisation' (page 36). To do this the Nursing and Care Quality Forum (2012) report to the government reinforced the need for leaders of organisations to ensure appropriate staffing levels and skills mix are in place and also highlighted the importance of leaders being supernumerary for them to be fully accountable and have the time to lead.

Effective role modelling and the advancement of practice knowledge and skills

The practice environment is the most influential learning milieu. It is where values are 'taught and caught' as well as skills learned, reinforced and practised. There is an increas-ing need to support less experienced nurses and health-care workers in order to ensure that the quality of learning, not only of knowledge and skills but also of caring attitudes, is given high priority. In Chapter 6, we used work by Noddings (2002) to discuss the impact of role modelling in the development of ethical caring. She asserted that our behaviour towards others could bring out the best or the worst in them and therefore helping people improve depended upon excellent role models. 'Whether I can become and remain a caring person – one who enters regularly in caring relations – depends in large part on how you respond to me' (page 15).

There is a strong call for more attention to be given to the recruitment of nursing stu-dents who can demonstrate that they are caring individuals, recruited for their caring nature and compassion as well as their knowledge and skills (Department of Health, 2012). Although this is commendable, sadly there is also some evidence that health-care students have to rethink their notions of caring soon after they enter the professions, and this questioning of their fundamental beliefs causes them uncertainty and doubt (Clouder, 2005). This could be related to unrealistic expectations but also because of the demanding nature of health care, emotional and physical, in which they need not only support but positive role models to emulate. Entry into a culture of caring is therefore very likely to have positive implications for nurse retention, not only for students but also for qualified nurses. Maben *et al.* (2007) described frustration and 'burn-out' experienced by newly registered nurses as they found they were unable to provide what they most wanted to give: patient-centred, holistic care. The authors found that this led to 'job-hopping' and in some cases a decision to leave the profession. However, in another study of newly qualified community nurses, a good role model early on, as part of a supportive induction process, if only for a short period of time, was shown to be beneficial and could influence growth in self-confidence, enabling the nurses to work independently and integrate into the community team (Brigham *et al.*, 2011).

Role models are important in the advancement of caring practice knowledge and skills by being examples to others who are likely to emulate them. They can not only help other nurses to incorporate appropriate values and attitudes but enable them to discover nursing knowledge embedded in clinical practice. They can also be important in participating in and promoting evidence-based practice and research . The skills of coaching, facilitating and role modelling are all necessary for effective mentorship, preceptorship, clinical supervision and appraisal.

Effective mentorship, preceptorship and clinical supervision

The value of these roles within clinical practice is recognised but at times of pressure may not be given high priority. If they are not implemented systematically, sensitively and knowledgeably, they can cause frustration, despondency and have negative consequences. Firth-Cozens and Cornwell (2009) highlight the difficulty with 'bad role models' who may exert powerful influences on the attitudes and behaviours of others. We know that if caring communities are to be built up and sustained, individuals need to be supported, developed and challenged. Good mentors, preceptors and supervisors will do just this and they need therefore to be recognised and valued as essential to compassionate care. Assessors also have an important part to play. This was noted by the Nursing and Care Quality Forum (2012), who indicated that managers should build the assessment of appropriate values into their ongoing supervision and development systems (including their annual appraisal process).

It would therefore seem that supportive structures such as these have the potential to promote caring if adequate training is provided, they are implemented systematically, and contain clear guidelines for those in a supervisory role and those being supervised. Evaluations need to be aimed at monitoring their effectiveness in relation to what they add to the development of the individual and to the culture of caring within the working environment.

Ensuring a caring environment in which fundamental as well as advanced needs are met

As we have seen in our discussion of what caring means to service users and their families, meeting fundamental needs is vitally important in demonstrating that we do care, that we prevent unnecessary pain and discomfort, nutritional deficiencies and other complications. The caring indicators demonstrated that even the smallest act of kindness has an impact on patient experience and the confidence service users and their families may have in service provision. In the 'Confidence in Caring' project (Department of Health, 2008) five 'confidence creators' were identified: a calm, clean, safe environment; a positive, friendly culture; good teamworking and good relationships; well-managed care with efficient delivery; and personalised care for and about every patient. The project provides a useful framework against which confidence in caring can be measured.

We have argued that although there is much evidence of good care the importance, value and impact of some caring approaches have not been understood, measured or given enough attention in everyday practice, whether in hospital or community care situations. It seems it is often only when caring is missing that it is noticed by the public and the press and becomes the focus for discussion and action. It could be that nurses are in danger of becoming so focused on expanding or advancing roles and meeting the demands of complex organisational requirements that less attention has been given to their role in understanding the importance of monitoring overall care. Important aspects of care are often delegated to other health-care workers but it is the nurse who has the responsibility for the appropriateness of the delegation and is accountable for the quality of the care undertaken. The NMC Code of Conduct (2008;29-31) requires that nurses and midwives must:

+ establish that anyone they delegate to is able to carry out their instructions;
+ confirm that the outcome of any delegated task meets required standards;
+ make sure that everyone who is delegated is supervised and supported.

Incorporating ethical, legal and professional guidelines and requirements

In their professional relationships with members of the public, what they do with them and for them, nurses must be guided by various ethical and legal frameworks, standards, policies and procedures. For example, the Mental Health Act (Department of Health, 2007) sets out clear legal requirements for caring for people with mental health problems, and nurses working with children and their families need to be aware of legislation related to safeguarding children. An example of guidance is the NHS Constitution, which establishes the principles and values of the NHS and pledges its commitments. It sets out the rights and responsibilities that public, patients and staff 'owe to one another' to ensure that the NHS operates fairly and effectively (Department of Health, 2012). Therefore, to be fair and effective in practice, nurses need up-to-date knowledge of various legal requirements, including those related to anti-discriminatory practice and the resources required to implement this.

The NMC Code of Conduct is a key tool for safeguarding the health and well-being of the public. It is about being professional, about being accountable, and about being able to justify decisions (NMC, 2008). However although legal requirements are mandatory, as the Confidence in Caring report states (Department of Health, 2008:5), standards, policies and competencies only guarantee what people can do, not what they do in practice. As we have seen from our stories, there are many ethical dilemmas in practice and although the Code is very helpful, it is also through knowledge gained from academic and practice sources that compassionate caring decisions can be made. Throughout this text, the caring indicators demonstrate that we have to use learning from a wide variety of sources, including academic, legal and ethical frameworks, and professional guidelines, but also from patients and their carers, colleagues and nursing research. Compassionate caring therefore requires an ongoing commitment to professional development and lifelong learning.

Evidence of effective partnerships with service users, other professionals and agencies

Throughout the text we have identified the importance of effective partnerships. We have emphasised the importance of working with others including patients and their families, listening to their 'lived experiences' and learning from them.

In addition other new ways of working are called for as traditional ways are insufficient if nurses are to be at the forefront of delivering high-quality compassionate care. Nurses need to expand their expertise in working with professionals and other agencies. For example, Stuart (2012) describes the importance of this for nurses in working in child care where they need to build relationships with numerous and varied organisations. Collaborations such as these are expanding in all aspects of health and social care. Work by Edwards (2005) discusses the notion of 'relational agency', which describes the way in which building relationships and working with others across the workforce and accessing their distributed expertise can strengthen responsive actions to complex challenges. To collaborate effectively entails the development of a great deal of trust on the part of all team members and what Edwards sees as including not only knowing how and what, but also knowing who. This means nurses must have confidence in articulating what they can provide, be resilient, creative and flexible in order to deliver with others the effective services people want and need.

The value of nursing as emotional and social capital

Nurses are paid to provide care and other services, for which the taxpayer makes a large investment, and the importance of the work that they undertake has been demonstrated (DoH, 2010). The term 'capital' is used in economics and management to define the assets, resources and relative wealth of a particular group or commodity.

As we have seen, there are calls for a shift in emphasis away from a bio-medical or technical model towards a culture that recognises and 'gives due weight to the complexity of human dynamics and the human processes involved' (Firth-Cozens and Cornwell, 2009). It is heart-warming that there is increasing recognition of the importance of the value of what is described as 'emotional capital' in business management.

Goodrich (2012) describes a pilot study by the King's Fund to assess the effectiveness of Schwartz Center Rounds first implemented in the USA. Multidisciplinary staff meet once a month to discuss and reflect on emotional and social challenges associated with their work. Although still in its early stages, findings are positive in that the Rounds were said to have helped increase respect, empathy and understanding between staff. It was also found that by providing a forum where people could meet and discuss as equals, although in different roles and at different levels of seniority they were perceived as useful for building and supporting shared values and a caring organisation.

Gendron (2004), an economist and expert in human resources, considers that emotional capital involves emotional competencies within individuals, which are necessary for personal, professional and also for organisational development. She also suggests that these competencies are vital for social and economic success and therefore asserts that emotional capital must be taken into account seriously by policymakers, practitioners and business organisations. She explains it this way:

'Emotional capital is the set (resource) of emotional competencies which gives individuals and organizations the ability to use emotions to help individuals at solving problems and living a more effective life and the organization at facing economic and social changes and being successful and surviving in the new economics world . . . It is the head

working with the heart and the hands ... For a full and ethical use of Human Resource with a big H, that implies taking into account the three Hs of each individual: Hands, Head and Heart.' (Gendron, 2004:31)

What she is saying is important for us in that the emotional capital of the caring nurse is an important resource that needs to recognised, nurtured and developed. The notion of emotional capital as an important resource in the 'hard-nosed' business world reinforces the importance of perceiving compassionate caring as an asset. Nurses should be proud of the emotional support they give to others (service users, relatives or colleagues) and it should be recognised, developed and valued within the organisation. Emotional work is demanding and influential. If you continue to value the emotional work that you do – for yourself and others, you will use strategies that encourage and nurture this. By doing so you will enhance your working environment and help create a culture of compassionate caring.

Summary

The nature of nursing work gives us a valid reason to interact with patients and their families. Caring is not unique to nursing but a nurse's presence during periods when someone is feeling most vulnerable provides unique opportunities for compassionate care. There will be an important challenge for nurses in the future, as they struggle to retain caring relationships within organisations that are increasingly outcome-driven and have considerable economic constraints upon them. They have to develop their skills in providing and presenting a wide range of evidence concerning the difference that their caring skills make to the experiences of service users and also to the outcomes of their care. These are important aspects for all nurses, but particularly those with roles in leadership, management and research.

Nurses constantly face new challenges. In considering all the aspects required to meet these, nurses need to have confidence in their professional values, knowledge and skills so that, with others, they can help shape current and future care provision.

Nursing has an exciting future as it responds to the changing nature of health and social care to meet changing demographic trends and service user needs and expectations. There will continue to be a crossing-over of traditional professional boundaries and a blurring between health and social care. Nurses need to respond effectively and creatively to these changes but must also have the determination to keep compassionate caring at the very heart of nursing whatever the future brings.

Activity

Think of ways in which you will endeavour to keep compassionate caring at the heart of your practice. This may mean looking back (such as by using a reflective journal), but also looking forward. For example, think of ways in which care can be planned to truly reflect effective partnerships with patients and their carers. This could be whether you are working within your own discipline or with multi-professional or multi-agency colleagues.

References

Brigham, L, Maxwell, C and Smith, A (2012) Leading in practice: a case study of how health visitors share and develop good practice. *Community Practitioner*, 85, 5, 24-28.

Clouder, L (2005) Caring as a 'threshold concept': transforming students in higher education into health(care) professionals. *Teaching Higher Education* 10, 4, 505-517.

Department of Health (2008) *Confidence in Caring: a framework for best practice.* Available at **www.dh.gov.uk/publications** (last accessed 30/05/2012).

Department of Health (2009) *NHS 2010-2015: from good to great: preventative, people-centred, productive.* London: Stationery Office.

Department of Health (2010) *Front Line Care Report.* Available at: **http://webarchive .nationalarchives.gov.uk/20100331110400/http:/cnm.independent.gov.uk/** (last accessed 4/06/2012).

Department of Health (2012*) Nursing and Care Quality Forum.* Available at **http://www .dh.gov.uk/health/2012/04/nursing-quality/** (last accessed 5/06/2012).

Edwards, A (2005) Relational agency: learning to be a resourceful practitioner. *International Journal of Educational Research*; 43:168-82.

Firth-Cozens, J and Cornwell, J (2009) *The Point of Care; enabling compassionate care in acute hospital settings.* London: King's Fund.

Foster, T and Hawkins, J (2005) The therapeutic relationship: dead or merely impeded by technology. *British Journal of Nursing* **14,** 13, 698-702.

Gendron, B (2004) *Why emotional capital matters in education and in labour? Toward an optimal exploitation of human capital and knowledge management.* Les Cahiers de la Maison des Sciences Economiques, série rouge, n° 113. Paris Université Panthéon-Sorbonne.

Goodrich, J and Cornwell, J (2008) *Seeing the person in the patient: Point of Care Review Paper.* London: Kings Fund.

Goodrich, J (2012) Supporting hospital staff to provide compassionate care: Do Schwartz Center Rounds work in English hospitals? *Journal of Royal Society of Medicine* (JRSM) 105,3, 117-122. Available at: **http://jrsm.rsmjournals.com/content/105/3/117.** full (last accessed 05/06/2012).

Health Foundation (2011) *Annual Review 2011.* Available at: **www.health.org.uk/public/ cms/75/76/313/3371/Annual%20Review%202011.pdf?realName=CVRy3L.pdf** (last accessed 5/06/2012).

King's Fund Commission (2011) *The Future of Leadership and Management in the NHS. No more heroes report.* London: King's Fund.

Longley, M, Shaw, C and Dolan, G (2007) Nursing: Towards 2015. *Alternative scenarios for healthcare, nursing and nurse education in the UK in 2015.* Welsh Institute for Health and Social Care, University of Glamorgan.

Maben, J, Latter, S and Macleod Clark, J (2007) The sustainability of ideals, values and the nursing mandate: evidence from a longitudinal qualitative study. *Nursing Inquiry* 14, 2, 99-113.

Maben, J and Griffiths, P (2008) *Nurses in Society: starting the debate.* King's College, London. National Nursing Research Unit. Available at **www.kcl.ac.uk/content/1/ c6/04/32/16/NursesinsocietyFinalreport.pdf** (last accessed 05/06/2012).

Maxwell, C, Brigham, L, Logan J and Smith, A (2011) Challenges facing newly qualified community nurses: a qualitative study. *British Journal of Community Nursing* **16**, 6, 282-287.

Mishler, E (1991) *"Once upon a time...".* Journal of Narrative and Life History 2, 3, 101-108. Tschudin, V (1999) *Nurses Matter: Reclaiming our professional identity.* Basingstoke: Macmillan.

NMC (2008) *The code: Standards of conduct, performance and ethics for nurses and midwives.* London: NMC.

Noddings, N (2002) *Educating moral people: a caring alternative to character education.* New York: Teachers College Press.

Stuart, K (2012) Leading multi-professional teams in children's workforce: an action research project. *International Journal of Integrated Care.* Available at: **www.ijic.org** (last accessed 5/06/2012).